THE PSYCHIATRIC INTERVIEW
A PRACTICAL GUIDE

D1334622

Praise for *The Psychiatric Interview*

Straightforward, practical, and wise, yet often lighthearted and funny, a breath of fresh air . . . brims with extraordinary gifts . . . this book is alive, a remarkable achievement.

Leston Havens, M.D.
Professor of Psychiatry
Harvard Medical School
Cambridge, Massachusetts

If I had to choose one book to place into the hands of every p chiatric resident as they began interviewing patients, this wc be that book . . . offers almost as much to seasoned clinicia to beginners.

John B. Herman, N
Director of Adult Residency Traini
Massachusetts General Hospital and McLean Hospit
Boston, Massachusetts

An extremely valuable resource for graduate students, psychiatry residents, and psychology interns . . . warm and engaging writing style . . . covers a remarkable array of topics clearly and succinctl

Robert T. Muller, Ph.D., C.Psy
Assistant Professor of Psychol
York Univer
Toronto, Ontario, Car

THE PSYCHIATRIC INTERVIEW
A PRACTICAL GUIDE

Daniel J. Carlat, M.D.

Section Chief
Department of Psychiatry
Anna Jaques Hospital
Newburyport, Massachusetts

Practical Guides in Psychiatry

Daniel J. Carlat, M.D.
Series Editor

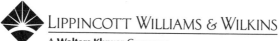

LIPPINCOTT WILLIAMS & WILKINS
A **Wolters Kluwer** Company
Philadelphia · Baltimore · New York · London
Buenos Aires · Hong Kong · Sydney · Tokyo

Acquisitions Editor: Charles W. Mitchell
Managing Editor/Developmental Editor: Frances M. Klass
Production Manager: Liane Carita
Supervising Editor: Mary Ann McLaughlin
Cover Designer: Jeane Norton
Production Editor: Allison Spearman, Silverchair Science +
    Communications
Compositor: Silverchair Science + Communications
Indexer: Elizabeth Willingham, Silverchair Science + Communications

Printed in the United States of America

09 8 7 6 5 4 3

Library of Congress Cataloging-in-Publication Data
Carlat, Daniel J.
    The psychiatric interview : a practical guide / Daniel J. Carlat.
        p.   cm.
    Includes bibliographical references and index.
    ISBN 0-683-30735-5
    1. Interviewing in psychiatry--Handbooks, manuals, etc.
2. Interviewing in psychiatry--Technique--Handbooks, manuals, etc.
3. Psychotherapist and patient--Handbooks, manuals, etc. I. Title.
    [DNLM: 1. Interview. Psychological--methods. 2. Mental Disorders-
-diagnosis. 3. Physician-Patient Relations. WM 141 C278p 1999]
RC480.7.C315 1999
616.89'075--dc21
DNLM/DLC
for Library of Congress   98-44274
                                                            CIP

To Tammy Bottner, my wife, soulmate, and teacher,
whose emotional and intellectual nurturance
allowed this book to see the light of day.

Acknowledgments

First, I thank Dr. Shawn Shea, without whose classic textbook, *Psychiatric Interviewing: The Art of Understanding*, and personal mentoring I would never have conceptualized this project.

Many members of the faculty of Massachusetts General Hospital (MGH), where I did my psychiatric residency, were extremely helpful in the shaping of the manuscript. In particular, I thank Dr. Ed Messner, whose very practical approach to patient care was refreshing; Dr. Paul Hamburg, who taught empathy and innumerable other aspects of connecting with patients; Dr. Paul Summergrad, a consummate clinician and the director of the inpatient unit during my chief residency, who supported me in my efforts to create an interviewing course for residents; Dr. Carey Gross, whose astonishing ability to rapidly make the right diagnosis for the most difficult patients is a continuing source of inspiration; and Dr. Anthony Erdmann, who generously contributed several screening questions.

Other MGH faculty who served as great teachers and mentors include Drs. John Herman, Kathy Sanders, Susan Skea, Ted Stern, Edie Gehringer, and Chris Gordon. In addition, special thanks go to Dr. Leston Havens, at the Cambridge Hospital, who was very encouraging throughout this project.

I also thank the psychiatry residents at MGH. The PGY-2 residents of the 1994 to 1995 academic year were extremely accommodating as I developed my interviewing curriculum while teaching it; the residents and psychology fellows in my own class constantly cheered me on, particularly Drs. Claudia Baldassano, Christina Demopulos, and Alan Lyman, co-members of the Harvard Gardens Club, and Dr. Robert Muller, psychologist supreme.

Finally, thanks are due to the staff of the Anna Jaques Hospital inpatient psychiatry unit, where I have been "road testing" the many techniques described in this book. I especially thank Dr. Rowen Hochstedler, my medical director, who is living proof that excellent mentoring can continue far beyond the reaches of academia.

Foreword

The Psychiatric Interview is straightforward, practical, and wise, yet often light-hearted and funny, a breath of fresh air where comparable references have often been boring and ponderous. It brims with extraordinary gifts for its readers. It is a scholarly review of the research literature, yet it moves swiftly and has a light, even jaunty, tone. It is very much up-to-date and serves as a useful introduction to many ideas, such as those from psychodynamics, that are not widely available to contemporary students.

Best of all, the book is alive, an extraordinary achievement in view of the amount of detailed material presented. It emphasizes the *person within the patient* and the need to form an *alliance* with that person to secure reliable information and cooperation in treatment. We *feel* the patients presented by Dr. Carlat; they are not simply diagnoses. Dr. Carlat offsets the profession's reputation for being cheerless and pathology-minded; he illustrates many ways by which effective relationships can be formed and shows how relationships that are endangered can be repaired, perhaps especially at the close of an interview.

The Psychiatric Interview is designed in an easily accessible format, with aids for memory, appendixes for organizing information, and sensible guides for recordkeeping. This is teaching by example at its best, with the examples both vivid and pointed, so that they stick in the reader's mind.

Truly understanding another human being is a daunting challenge, yet nothing is more important if we are to soothe the suffering of a ravaged soul. Use this book as a guide to reach for that understanding.

Leston Havens, M.D
Professor of Psychiatry
Harvard Medical School
The Cambridge Health Alliance
Cambridge, Massachusetts

Introduction

Over the course of a 40-year professional career, you will do approximately 100,000 diagnostic interviews. The diagnostic interview is by far the most important tool in the arsenal of any clinician, and yet the average training program directs relatively few resources to specific training in the skills required for it. The general assumption seems to be that if you do enough interviews with different kinds of patients, you'll naturally pick up the required skills. That may be true, but it can take a long time, and the learning process can be painful.

I hatched the idea for this manual one night during my first year of psychiatric residency. Starting my shift in the acute psychiatry service (APS), I noticed five patients in the waiting room; the resident who handed me the emergency room beeper said there were two more patients in the emergency room, both in restraints. At that moment the beeper sounded, and I called the number. "Psychiatry? This is Ellison 6. We have a patient up here who says he's depressed and suicidal. Please come and evaluate, STAT." That meant that I had a total of eight diagnostic assessments to do.

As the night stretched on, my interviews got briefer. The developmental history was the first to go, followed quickly by the formal mental status examination. This trimming process continued until, at 5 a.m., it reached its absurd, but inevitable, conclusion. My entire interview consisted of little more than the following question: "Are you suicidal?"

As I handed the beeper off to my colleague at 8 a.m. (I had slept for 50 minutes, about the length of a psychotherapeutic hour), I began to think about those interviews. Were they too short? (I was sure they were.) Were they efficient? (I doubted it.) Had anyone come up with a system for conducting diagnostic assessments that were rapid but at the same time thorough enough to do justice to the patient?

Looking for such a system became my little project over the rest of my residency. I labeled a manila file folder *interviewing pearls* and started throwing in bits and pieces of information from various sources, including interviewing textbooks, lectures in our Wednesday seminars, and conversations with my supervisors and with other residents. When I became chief resident of the inpatient unit, I videotaped case conferences and took notes on nice interviewing techniques. Later, during my first job as an attending psychiatrist, I practiced and fine-tuned these techniques with inpatients at Anna Jaques Hospital and outpatients at Harris Street Associates.

What I ended up with was a compendium of tips and pearls that will help make your diagnostic interviews more efficient and, I hope, more fun. Mnemonics will make it easier for you to quickly remember needed information. Interviewing techniques will help you move the interview along quickly without alienating your patients. Every chapter begins with an Essential Concepts box that lists the truly take-home items of information therein. The appendixes contain useful little stocking stuffers, such as "pocket cards" with vital information to be photocopied and forms that you can use during your interviews to ensure that you're not forgetting anything important.

However, if you're looking for theoretical justifications and point-by-point evidence for the efficacy of these techniques, you won't find it here. Go to one of the many textbooks of psychiatric interviewing for that. Every piece of information in this manual had to meet the following stringent standard: It had to be immediately useful knowledge for the trainee about to step into the room with a new patient.

WHAT THIS MANUAL *IS*

First, this is *only* a manual. It's not a residency or an internship. The way to learn how to interview patients is by interviewing them under good supervision. Only there can you learn the subtleties of the interview, the skills of understanding the interactions between you and your patients.

It is a tool that lends you a guiding hand in your initial efforts to interview patients. It's confusing territory. There are lots of mistakes to be made and many embarrassing and awkward moments ahead. This book won't prevent all of that, but it will catalyze the development of your interviewing skills.

It is a handbook for any beginning clinician who does psychiatric assessments as part of his or her training. This includes psychiatric residents, medical students, psychology interns, social work interns, mental health workers, nursing students, and residents in other medical fields who may need to do an on-the-spot diagnostic assessment while waiting for a consultant.

WHAT THIS MANUAL IS *NOT*

It is not a *textbook* of psychiatric interviewing. There are a number of interviewing textbooks already available (Shea 1988; Othmer 1994; Morrison 1995), my favorite being Shea's *Psychiatric Interviewing: The Art of Understanding*. Although textbooks are more thorough and encyclopedic, the drawback is that they do not guide the beginner to the essence of what he or she needs to know. Also, textbooks aren't portable, and I wanted to write something that you can carry around to your various clinical settings. That said, please buy a textbook, and have it around for those times when you want to read in more depth.

This is also not a handbook of psychiatric *disorders*. There are plenty of good ones already published, and I wrote this manual to fill the need for a brief, how-to guide to diagnosing those disorders.

Finally, it is not a *psychotherapy* manual. Doing a rapid diagnostic assessment isn't psychotherapy, although you can extend many of the skills used in the first interview to psychotherapy.

I hope that you will enjoy this book and that it will help you to develop confidence in interviewing. As you embark, remember these words of Theodore Roosevelt: "The only man who never makes a mistake is the man who never does anything." Good luck!

Contents

THE PSYCHIATRIC INTERVIEW
A PRACTICAL GUIDE

GENERAL PRINCIPLES OF EFFECTIVE INTERVIEWING

The most tactful question in the world is still inquisitive and requests an answer. To some measure, it carries the memory of all questions that could not be answered or were shaming or damning to acknowledge.

Leston Havens, M.D.
A Safe Place

The Initial Interview: A Preview

1

The Four Tasks
- Build a therapeutic alliance.
- Obtain the psychiatric database.
- Interview for diagnosis.
- Negotiate a treatment plan with your patient.

The Three Phases
- Opening phase.
- Body of the interview.
- Closing phase.

FOUR TASKS OF THE DIAGNOSTIC INTERVIEW

The diagnostic interview is really about treatment, not diagnosis. It's important to keep this larger goal in mind during the interview, because if you don't, your patient may never return for a second visit, and your finely wrought *Diagnostic and Statistical Manual of Mental Disorders, Fourth Edition* (*DSM-IV*) diagnosis will end up languishing in a chart in a file room.

Studies show that up to 50% of patients drop out before the fourth session of treatment, and many never return after the first appointment (Baekeland and Lundwall 1975). The reasons for treatment dropout are many. Some patients do not return because they formed poor alliances with their clinicians, some because they weren't really interested in treatment in the first place, and others because the initial interviews alone boosted their morale enough to get them through their stressors (Pekarik 1993). The upshot is that much more than diagnosis should occur during the initial interview: Alliance building, morale boosting, and treatment negotiating are also vital.

The four tasks of the initial interview blend with one another. You establish a therapeutic alliance as you learn about your patient. The very act of inquiry is an alliance builder; we tend to like people who are warmly curious about us. As you ask questions, you formulate possible diagnoses, and thinking through diagnoses leads naturally to the process of negotiating a treatment plan.

Build a Therapeutic Alliance

A therapeutic alliance forms the groundwork of any psychological treatment. Chapter 3, The Therapeutic Alliance, focuses on the alliance directly, and Chapters 4 to 10 provide various interviewing tips that will help you increase rapport with your patient.

Obtain the Psychiatric Database

Also known as the *psychiatric history*, the psychiatric database includes historical information relevant to the current clinical presentation. These topics are covered in Part II, The Psychiatric History, and include history of present illness (HPI), psychiatric history, medical history, family psychiatric history, and aspects of the social and developmental history. Gleaning this information is the substance of the interview, and throughout this step you will have to work on building and maintaining the alliance. You will also make frequent forays into the next task, interviewing for diagnosis.

Interview for Diagnosis

The ability to interview for diagnosis—without sounding as if you're reading off a checklist of symptoms and without getting sidetracked by less relevant information—is one of the supreme skills of a clinician, and one that you will hone and develop over the course of your professional life. Part III, Interviewing for Diagnosis, is devoted to this skill; it contains chapters on how to memorize *DSM-IV* criteria (Chapter 17) and on the art of diagnostic hypothesis testing (Chapter 18) and several disorder-specific chapters that focus on how to use screening and probing questions for each of the major *DSM-IV* disorders (Chapters 21 to 28).

Negotiate a Treatment Plan and Communicate It to Your Patient

This process is rarely taught in residency or graduate school, and yet it is probably the most important thing you can do to ensure that your patient adheres to whatever treatment you recommend. If your patient doesn't understand your formulation, doesn't agree with your advice, and doesn't feel comfortable telling you so, the interview may as well never have taken place. See Part IV, Interviewing for Treatment, for tips on the art of patient education and clinical negotiation.

THREE PHASES OF THE DIAGNOSTIC INTERVIEW

The diagnostic interview, like most tasks in life, has a beginning, a middle, and an end. Although this may seem obvious enough, novice interviewers often lose sight of it and therefore fail to actively structure the interview and control its pacing. The result is usually a panic-filled ending, in which 50 questions are wedged into the last 5 minutes.

It's true that there's a huge amount of information to obtain during the first interview, and time may feel like the enemy. Excellent interviewers, however, rarely feel rushed. They have the ability to obtain large amounts of information in a brief period, without giving patients the sense that they are being hurried along or made to fit into a preordained structure. One of the secrets of a good interviewer is the ability to actively structure the interview in its three phases.

Opening Phase (5 to 10 minutes)

The opening phase includes meeting your patient, learning a bit about her life situation, and then shutting up and giving her a few uninterrupted minutes to tell you why she came. This is discussed in more detail in Chapter 3, because the opening phase is a crucial period for alliance building; the patient is making an initial decision as to your trustworthiness. The opening phase is based on careful, preinterview preparation, covered in Chapter 2, Logistic Preparations: What to Do Before the Interview. Attention to logistics ensures that you will be completely attuned to the relationship with your patient during the first 5 minutes.

Body of the Interview (30 to 40 minutes)

Over the course of the opening phase, you will come up with some initial diagnostic hypotheses (Chapter 18), and you will decide on some interviewing priorities to explore during the body of the interview. For example, you may decide that depression, anxiety, and substance abuse are likely problems for a particular patient. You will map out an interviewing strategy for exploring these topics, which will include asking about the history of the present illness (Chapter 12); history of depression, suicidal ideation (SI), and substance abuse (Chapters 20, 21, and 24); family history of these disorders (Chapter 15); and a detailed assessment of whether the patient actually meets *DSM-IV* criteria (Chapters 20, 21, and 24) for each disorder. Once you've accomplished these priority tasks, you can move on to other topics, such as the social/developmental history (Chapter 16), medical history (Chapter 14), and psychiatric review of symptoms (PROS) (Part III).

Closing Phase (5 to 10 minutes)

Although you may be tempted to continue asking diagnostic questions right up to the end of the hour, it's essential to reserve at least 5 minutes for the closing phase of the interview. The closing phase should include two components: (a) a discussion of your assessment, using the patient education techniques outlined in Chapter 29 and (b) an effort to come to a negotiated agreement about treatment or follow-up plans (Chapter 30). Of course, early in your career it will be difficult to come up with a coherent assessment on the spot, without the benefit of hours of postinterview supervision and reading. This skill will improve with practice.

2 Logistic Preparations: What to Do before the Interview

Essential Concepts
- Prepare the right space and time.
- Use paper tools effectively.
- Develop your policies.

The work of psychological healing begins in a safe place, to be compared with the best of hospital experience or, from an earlier time, church sanctuary. The psychological safe place permits the individual to make spontaneous, forceful gestures and, at the same time, represents a community that both allows the gestures and is valued for its own sake.

Leston Havens, M.D.
A Safe Place

Logistic preparation for an interview is important because it sets up a mellower and less stressful experience for both you and your patient. Often, trainees are thrown into the clinic without training in how to find and secure a room, how to deal with scheduling, or how to document effectively. You'll eventually arrive at a system that works well for you; this chapter will help speed up that process.

PREPARE THE RIGHT SPACE AND TIME

Secure a Space

A space war is raging in most clinics and training programs, and you must fight to secure territory. Once secured, dig trenches, call for the cavalry, do whatever you need to do.

I remember one early lesson in this reality: I was 2 months into my training and just finishing supervision in the Warren Building of the Massachusetts General Hospital (MGH) campus. It was 12:55 p.m., and I had a therapy patient scheduled for 1:00 p.m. in the Ambulatory Care Clinic, a building so far from Warren that it practically had its own time zone. I zigged and zagged around staff and patients in the hallways on their way to the cafeteria and rushed into the clinic by 1:05. My patient was in the waiting room and got a good view of sweat trickling down my forehead. I scanned the room schedule and found that no rooms were free. Panic set in, until the secretary pointed out that the resident who had room 825 for that hour had not yet shown up. So I led my patient to 825, and we started, 10 minutes late. Five minutes later, there was a knock on the door. I opened it, and there stood the resident and his patient. I redeposited my patient in the waiting room and scoured the list for another room.

I won't torture you with the rest of this saga. Suffice it to say we were evicted from the next room as well, and the therapy session was, in the end, only 15 minutes long, with much humiliation on my part and good-natured amusement on my patient's.

Here are some time-honored tips on how to secure a room and what to do with it once you have it:

- **Schedule the same time every week.** Try to secure your room for the same time every week. That way you'll be able to fit interviews into your weekly schedule routinely. When it comes to psychiatric interviewing, routine is your friend. Psychodynamic psychotherapists call this routine—the same time, the same room, the same greeting—the "frame." Making it invariable reduces distractions from the work of psychological exploration.

- **Make your room your own in some way.** This isn't easy when you only inhabit it for a few hours a week. Clinic policy may forbid this, or it may be impolite (e.g., if you're using an office that belongs to a regular staff member). If possible, put a picture on the desk or the wall, bring a plant in, place some reference books on a shelf, hang some files. The room will feel more like your space, and it will seem homier to your patient. By the way, if you do put up a picture, think twice before you display your friends or family; it may lead to transference problems with some patients.

- **Arrange the seating so that you can see a clock** without shifting your gaze too much. A wall clock positioned just behind your patient works well. A desk clock or a wristwatch placed between the two of you is also acceptable. The object is to allow you to keep track of the passage of time without this being obvious to your patient. It is alienating for a patient to notice a clinician frequently looking at a clock; the perceived message is "I can't wait for the end of this interview." You do need to monitor the time, though, to ensure that you obtain a tremendous amount of information in a brief period. Actually, keeping track of time will paradoxically make you *less* distracted and *more* present for your patient, since you'll always know that you're managing your time adequately.

Protect Your Time

Time is but the stream I go a-fishing in.

Henry David Thoreau

This is not to say that you should go fly-casting with your patients (though you're usually fishing for something or other during an interview). Rather, you should protect the time you schedule for interviews so that it has that same peaceful, almost sacred quality. How to do it?

- **Arrive earlier than the patient.** You need time to prepare yourself emotionally and logistically for the interview. Compose yourself. Lay out whatever forms or handouts you'll need. Answer any urgent messages that you just picked up at your message box. Breathe, meditate, do a crossword puzzle or whatever you do to relax.

  I once observed an interviewer who was visibly anxious. He crossed and uncrossed his legs and constantly kneaded his left palm with his right thumb. Eventually the patient interrupted the interview and asked, "Doctor? Are you all right? You look nervous." He laughed. "Oh, I'm fine," he said. And no, this was not a resident, but one of my professors.

- **Prevent interruptions.** There are various ways to prevent interruptions:

  Ask the clinic secretary to take messages for you.

  Ask the page operator to hold all but urgent pages.

  Put your pager on vibrate mode and only answer urgent pages.

  Sign your pages out to a colleague.

- **Don't overbook patients.** Know your limits. At the beginning, it may take you an hour and a half to complete an evaluation, not including the write-up. If so, book only one patient per 2-hour slot. Obviously, your training program won't allow you to maintain such a leisurely schedule for long, but you will improve and become more efficient. Eventually, you should aim toward completing the evaluation and write-up (or dictation) in 1 hour.

- **Leave plenty of time for notes and paperwork.** The time required for paperwork will vary, depending on both the setting and the clinician. The key is to figure out how long it takes you and then to make room for it in your schedule. Don't fall into denial. If you happen to be very slow at paperwork, admit it and plan accordingly.

I know an excellent psychiatrist who has learned from experience that he has to spend thirty minutes on charting, telephoning, and miscellaneous paperwork related to patients for every hour of clinical work he does. If he spends 6 hours seeing patients, he schedules 3 hours in the evening to take care of the collateral work. Although his hourly wage decreases, he gains the satisfaction of knowing that he's doing the kind of job he wants to do.

Now, that wouldn't work for me. I schedule slightly less time with patients so that I can finish all collateral work before I see my next appointment. The point, as Polonius said in *Hamlet*, is to "Know thyself, and to thine own self be true."

USE PAPER TOOLS EFFECTIVELY

By "paper tools," I mean the whole array of interview forms, cheat-sheets, patient handouts, and patient questionnaires. There's little formal training in how to use these, but they are indispensable when you see a lot of patients every day. All of the paper tools I discuss below are in the appendices of this manual, and you are welcome to copy and use what you want. You might find all, some, or none of them useful, or you may want to adapt them to better suit your needs.

Psychiatric Interview Long Form

This psychiatric interview long form (in Appendix B) is adapted from the one used by Anthony Erdmann, an attending psychiatrist at MGH. He takes notes on it while talking to patients and puts it in his chart.

Advantages.   Use of this form ensures a thorough data evaluation and saves time, because notes can be placed directly into the chart.

Disadvantages.   Some patients may be alienated if you seem more interested in completing a form than in getting to know them.

Psychiatric Interview Short Form

The short form (in Appendix B) can be used for rough notes when you are going to dictate the evaluation or write it up in a longer version later.

Advantages. This form presents less of a barrier between clinician and patient than the long form and is easy to refer to while dictating.

Disadvantages. Use of the short form may lead to a less thorough evaluation.

Psychiatric Interview Pocket Card

The pocket card (in Appendix A) is used to remind you of all the topics to cover. You can jot rough notes on a blank piece of paper or not take notes at all, if you're able to remember most information.

Advantages. The card allows maximum interaction between clinician and patient, since there is no form to fill out.

Disadvantages. Required information is not fully spelled out on the pocket card, so more use of memory is required.

Patient Questionnaire*

Some clinicians give their patients a questionnaire (in Appendix B) such as this one before the first meeting, to decrease the time needed to acquire basic information.

Advantages. The patient questionnaire allows more time during the first session to focus on issues of immediate concern to the patient. It may heighten the patient's sense that he is actively participating in his care.

Disadvantages. If all of the patient's answers on the questionnaire are accepted at face value, invalid information may be collected. Some patients may view filling out the questionnaire as a burden.

Patient Handouts

Patients usually appreciate receiving some written information (in Appendix C) about their disorder, and it probably increases treatment compliance.

---

*Adapted from the questionnaire of Edward Messner, M.D.

Advantages.   Patient handouts increase patients' understanding of their diagnosis and gives them a sense that they are collaborating in their treatment.

Disadvantages.   The handouts may present more information than some patients can handle early in their treatment. Information may also be misinterpreted.

DEVELOP YOUR POLICIES

From the first appointment with a particular patient, you are entering into a relationship. You need to determine the parameters of this relationship, including issues such as how and when you can be contacted, what the patient should do in case of an emergency, who *you* can talk to about the patient, and how to deal with missed appointments. As you face this array of decisions, the following tips and ideas should help you devise policies that fit your personality and clinical setting.

Contacting You

You define the boundaries of the clinical relationship by setting limits on where and when patients can reach you. Do this early on; if you don't, you'll eventually suffer for it.

I found this out the hard way with my very first therapy patient during residency. She was a 40-year-old woman I'll call Sally who had panic disorder and depression. I first met her in the crisis clinic, where she came after an upsetting conversation with her father. I spoke to her for half an hour, and I gave her a follow-up appointment for the next week—and I gave her my pager number and told her that this was a way to reach me, "anytime." The next Saturday morning, over breakfast and the paper, I got my first page: "Call Sally." She was in the middle of a panic attack, which subsided after a 10-minute conversation. Later that day, as I was riding my bike, I got another page . . . "Call Sally." I was somewhere on a country road in Concord, Massachusetts, and far from a phone. Ten minutes later: "Call Sally. Urgent." Over the next hour I received six pages, each sounding more urgent as the alarmed hospital operator added more and more punctuation. The last page read, "Call Sally!!! Emergency!!!!!!" When I finally found a pay phone, my heart pounding, Sally said, "Doctor! I just had another panic attack."

I felt the first hint of what I later learned was "counter-transference." At the time, I called it "being pissed off." I tried to keep the irritation out of my voice as I told her she didn't have to call me every time she had a panic attack. At our next appointment, after some good supervision, I laid out some ground rules. Sally could page me only during the week between 8 a.m. and 5 p.m. Otherwise, she was instructed to go to the crisis clinic. This in itself helped decrease the frequency of her panic attacks, since it took away the reinforcement of a phone conversation with her therapist every time she panicked.

Suggestions

- Never give your home telephone number to patients, and consider keeping an unlisted phone number.
- You may give out your paging number, but specify the times when you're available to be paged. Don't let your life revolve around your pager. Tell your patient what to do if there is an emergency at a time when you are *not* available for paging. For example, he can call the crisis clinic, and you can give the clinic instructions to page you after hours if the on-call clinician judges that the situation warrants your immediate involvement.
- If you have a voice-mail system, have patients reach you there. Your voice mail is accessible 24 hours a day, and you can check it whenever you want and decide who to call back and when. Some patients will call your voice mail just to be soothed by your recorded voice.
- When you're on vacation, I suggest you sign your patients out to a clinician you know and trust, rather than have them call the crisis clinic during regular hours. That way, you can ensure that someone is prepared to deal with any impending crises. For example, you may have patients who are chronically suicidal but rarely require hospitalization and can be managed through crises with frequent outpatient support. Letting your colleague know about these patients may prevent inappropriate hospitalization.

Contacting the Patient

Be sure to get your patient's various phone numbers (e.g., home, work, day treatment program). Ask whether it's okay for you to identify yourself when you call, because some patients don't want employers or family members to know that they're in treatment. Obtain numbers of family members or close friends so that you can contact them either to gather clinical information or in emergency situations. You'll need to obtain your patient's consent for this ahead of time.

Missed Appointments

The usual practice is to tell patients that they must inform you at least 24 hours in advance of any missed appointments or they will be charged, except in emergency situations. As a salaried trainee, the financial aspects of this policy aren't relevant, but there are important clinical benefits. Patients who make the effort to show up for sessions show a level of commitment that bodes well for therapeutic success. This policy encourages that commitment.

What if a patient repeatedly cancels sessions (albeit in time to avoid paying)? First, figure out why she is canceling. Is it for a legitimate reason, or is she acting out some feelings of anxiety or hostility? Did you just return from vacation? If so, this is a common time for patients to act out a sense of having been abandoned by you.

One way to approach this issue is head-on:

> *I notice that since I returned from vacation, you've canceled three sessions in a row. What's going on? Sometimes people get angry at their therapists.*

> *I've noticed that since we started talking about the causes of your bulimia, you've missed a lot of sessions. Should we be going a bit more slowly with these issues?*

The Therapeutic Alliance: What It Is, Why It's Important, and How to Establish It

> ## *Essential Concepts*
> - Be warm, courteous, and emotionally sensitive.
> - Actively defuse the strangeness of the clinical situation.
> - Give your patient the opening word.
> - Gain your patient's trust by projecting competence.

The therapeutic alliance is a feeling that you should create over the course of the diagnostic interview, a sense of rapport, trust, and warmth. Most research on the therapeutic alliance has been done in the context of psychotherapy, rather than the diagnostic interview. Jerome Frank, author of *Persuasion and Healing* (Frank 1991) and the father of the comparative study of psychotherapy, found that a therapeutic alliance is the most important ingredient in all effective psychotherapies. Creating rapport is truly an art and therefore difficult to teach, but here are some tips that should increase your success.

BE WARM, COURTEOUS, AND EMOTIONALLY SENSITIVE

Are there any specific interviewing techniques that lead to good rapport? Surprisingly, the answer appears to be "no," and that is good news. A group of researchers from London have studied this question in depth and published their results in seven papers in the *British Journal of Psychiatry* (Cox et al. 1981a, 1981b, 1988). Their bottom line was that several interviewing styles were equally effective in eliciting emotions. As long as the trainees whom they observed behaved with a basic sense of warmth, courtesy, and sensitivity, it didn't particularly matter which techniques they used; all techniques worked well.

No book can teach you warmth, courtesy, or sensitivity. These are attributes that you probably already have if you are in one of the helping professions. Just be sure to consciously activate these qualities during your initial interview.

There are, however, some specific rapport-building techniques that you should be aware of:

- **Empathic or sympathetic statements,** such as "you must have felt terrible when she left you," communicate your acceptance and understanding of painful emotions. Be careful not to overuse empathic statements, because they can sound wooden and insincere if forced.
- **Direct feeling questions,** such as "How did you feel when she left you?" are also effective.
- **Reflective statements,** such as "You sound sad when you talk about her," are effective but also should not be overused, because it can seem as though you are stating the obvious.

What do you do if you don't like your patient? Certainly, some patients immediately seem unlikeable, perhaps because of their anger, passivity, or dependence. If you are bothered by such qualities, it's often helpful to see them as expressions of psychopathology and awaken your compassion for the patient on that basis. It may also be that your negative feelings are expressions of countertransference, which is discussed in Chapter 11.

ACTIVELY DEFUSE THE STRANGENESS OF THE CLINICAL SITUATION

It's easy to lose sight of the fact that an hour-long psychiatric interview is a strange and anxiety-provoking experience. Your patient is expected to reveal his deepest and most shameful secrets to a perfect stranger. There are several ways to quickly defuse that strangeness.

- **Greet your patient naturally.** While there are many perfectly acceptable ways to greet patients, a general rule of thumb is to act naturally, which usually means introducing yourself and shaking hands. I often engage in some small talk for the first few seconds, because many patients have a distorted view of psychiatrists as mysterious, silent types who busily scrutinize a patient's smallest gestures. Small talk undermines this projection and puts the patient at ease. Acceptable topics include the weather and difficulties arriving at the office.

> *Hi, I'm Dr. Carlat. Nice to meet you. I hope you were able to make your way through the maze of the hospital without too much trouble.*

Ask the patient what he wants to be called, and make sure to use that name a few times during the interview.

> *Do you prefer that I call you Mr. Whalen, or Michael, or something else?*

Using the patient's name, especially the first name, is a great way of increasing a sense of familiarity.

▼ **Caveat:** Some patients (as well as some clinicians) view small talk as unprofessional. I try to size up my patient visually before deciding how to greet him. For example, small talk is rarely appropriate for patients who are in obvious emotional pain or for grossly psychotic patients, particularly if they are paranoid.

- **Get to know the patient as a person first.** Some patients find it awkward to reveal sensitive information to a stranger. If you sense that this is the case, you might want to begin by learning something about them as people.

> *Before we get into the issues that brought you here, I'd like to know a little bit about you as a person—where you live, what you do, that sort of thing.*

Learning a bit about your patient's demographics at the outset has the added advantage of helping you start your diagnostic hypothesizing. There's a reason why the standard opening line of a written or oral case presentation is a description of demographics: "This is a 75-year-old white widower who is a retired police officer and lives alone in a small apartment downtown." You can already begin to make diagnostic hypotheses: "He's a widower and thus at high risk for depression. He's elderly, so at higher risk for dementia. He apparently had a career as a police officer, so probably is not schizophrenic," and so on. Knowing basic demographics at the outset doesn't excuse you from asking all the questions required for a diagnostic evaluation, but it certainly helps set priorities in the direction of inquiry.

- **Educate the patient about the nature of the interview.** Not every patient understands the nature of an evaluation interview. Some may think that this is the first session in a long-term psychotherapy. They may come into the interview with the negative, media-fed expectation of a clinician who sits quietly and inscrutably while the patient pours out his soul. Others may have no idea why they are talking to you, having been referred to a "doctor" by an internist who believes psychological factors are interfering with their medical treatment. Thus, it's helpful to begin by asking the patient if he understands the purpose of the interview, and then to give him your explanation, including the expected length of time of the interview, what sorts of information you'll be asking about, and whether you will follow him for further treatment if needed.

> Interviewer (I): So, Mr. Johnson, did your doctor explain the purpose of this interview?
>
> Patient (P): She said you might be able to help me with my nerves.
>
> I: I certainly hope I can do that. This is what we call an evaluation interview. We'll be meeting for about 50 minutes today, and I'll be asking you all sorts of questions, some about your nerves, some about your family and other things, all so I can best understand what might be causing you the troubles you've been having. Depending on your problem, we may need to meet twice to complete this evaluation, but the way our clinic works is that I won't necessarily be the one who will treat you over the long term; depending on what I think is going on, I may refer you to someone else for treatment.

- **Address your patient's projections.** Keep in mind that a lot of shame is associated with psychiatric disorders. Patients commonly project aspects of their own negative self-images onto you. They may see you as critical or judgmental. Havens (1986) recognized this and encouraged the use of "counterprojective statements" to increase the patient's sense of safety:

> *It may be embarrassing for you to reveal all these things to a stranger. Who knows how I'd react? In fact, I'm here to understand you and to help you.*

CLINICAL VIGNETTE

Paranoid patients often project malevolent intentions onto the interviewer. In this example, the interviewer addresses these projections directly:

> I: *Are you concerned about why I'm asking all these questions?*
>
> P: *Sure. You've got to wonder—What's in it for you? How are you going to use all this information?*
>
> I: *I'm going to use it to understand you better and to help you. It won't go any further than this room.*
>
> P: *(Smirking) I've heard that before.*
>
> I: *Did someone turn it against you?*
>
> P: *You bet.*
>
> I: *Then I can understand that you'd be careful about talking to me—you probably think I'd do the same thing.*
>
> P: *You never know.*

With the distrust issue brought out into the open, the patient was more forthcoming throughout the rest of the interview.

GIVE YOUR PATIENT THE OPENING WORD

In one study of physicians, patients were allowed to complete their opening statements of concern in only 23% of cases (Beckman and Franckel 1984). An average of 18 seconds elapsed before these patients were interrupted. The consequence of this highly controlling interviewing style is that important clinical information may never make it out of the patient's mouth (Platt and McMath 1979).

You should allow your patients about 5 minutes of "free speech" (Morrison 1995) before you ask specific questions. This accomplishes two goals: First, it gives your patient the sense that you are interested in listening, thereby establishing rapport, and second, it increases the likelihood that you will understand the issues that are most troubling to the patient and thereby make a correct diagnosis. Shea (1988) has called this initial listening phase the "scouting period," because you can use it to scout for clues to psychopathology that you will want to follow up on later in the interview. It has also been called the "warm up" period by Othmer and Othmer (1994), because one of its purposes is to create a comfort level between you and the patient so that the patient is not put off by the large number of diagnostic questions to come.

Of course, you have to be flexible. Some patients begin in such a vague or disorganized fashion that you will have to ask your questions right away, whereas others are so articulate that if you let them talk for 10 or 20 minutes, they will tell you almost everything you need to know.

Each clinician develops his or her own first question, but all first questions should be open-ended and should invite the patient's story. Here are several examples of first questions:

> *What was it that brought you to the clinic today?*
>
> *What brings you to see me today?*
>
> *What sorts of things have been troubling you?*
>
> *How can I be of help to you?*
>
> *What can I do for you?*

GAIN YOUR PATIENT'S TRUST BY PROJECTING COMPETENCE

This is always a tricky issue for novice interviewers, who often feel anything but competent. In fact, your patient usually gives you the benefit of the doubt here, because of something called "ascribed" competence. This is the competence your patient attributes to you purely because of your institutional ties. You work for Hospital X or University Y, so you must be competent. Ascribed confidence will get you through the first several minutes of the interview, but after that, you have to earn your patient's respect.

Gaining a patient's trust is easier than you might think. Even as a novice, you know much more about mental illness than your patient, and this knowledge is communicated by the kinds of questions you ask. For example, your patient tells you she is depressed. You immediately ask questions about sleep and appetite. Most patients will be impressed by your ability to elicit relevant data in this way.

Other, more prosaic ways of projecting competence include dressing professionally and adopting a general attitude of confidence. At the end of the interview, your ability to provide meaningful feedback will further cement your patient's respect.

Asking Questions I: How to Approach Threatening Topics

Essential Concepts

- Use normalizing questions to decrease a patient's sense of embarrassment about a feeling or behavior.
- Use symptom expectation and reduction of guilt to defuse the admission of embarrassing behavior.
- Use symptom exaggeration to determine the actual frequency of a sensitive or shameful behavior.
- Use familiar language when asking about behaviors.

Always the beautiful answer who asks a more beautiful question.

e. e. cummings

Over the course of the diagnostic interview, many of your questions will be threatening to your patient. The simple admission of psychiatric symptoms is humiliating for many people, as is the admission of behaviors considered by society to be either undesirable or abnormal. Such behaviors include drug and alcohol abuse, violence, and homosexuality. Beyond this, there are other behaviors that your patients may not want to admit, because they may think you will disapprove of them personally. These might include a history of noncompliance with mental health treatment, a checkered work history, or a deficient social life.

To maintain a healthy self-image, patients may lie when asked what they perceive to be threatening questions. This has been a significant problem among both clinicians and professional surveyors for years, and a repertoire of interviewing techniques has been developed to increase the validity of responses to threatening questions (Payne 1951; Shea 1988; Sudman and Bradburn 1987). Good clinicians instinctively use many of these techniques, having found through trial and error that they improve the validity of the interview.

NORMALIZATION

Normalization is the most common and useful technique for eliciting sensitive or embarrassing material. The technique involves introducing your question with some type of normalizing statement. There are two principal ways to do this:

1. Start the question by implying that the behavior is a normal or understandable response to a mood or situation:

   With all the stress you've been under, I wonder if you've been drinking more lately?

   Sometimes when people are very depressed, they think of hurting themselves. Has this been true for you?

   Sometimes when people are under stress or are feeling lonely, they binge on large amounts of food to make themselves feel better. Is this true for you?

2. Begin by describing another patient (or patients) who has engaged in the behavior, showing your patient that she is not alone:

   I've seen a number of patients who've told me that their anxiety causes them to avoid doing things, like driving on the highway or going to the grocery store. Has that been true for you?

   I've talked to several patients who've said that their depression causes them to have strange experiences, like hearing voices or thinking that strangers are laughing at them. Has that been happening to you?

It's possible to go too far with normalization. Some behaviors are impossible to consider normal or understandable, such as acts of extreme violence or sexual abuse, so don't use normalization to ask about these.

SYMPTOM EXPECTATION

Symptom expectation, also known as the "gentle assumption" (Shea 1988), is similar to normalization: You communicate that a behavior is in some way normal or expected. Phrase your questions to imply that you already assume the patient has engaged in some behavior and that you will not be offended by a positive response. This technique is most useful when you have a high index of suspicion of some self-destructive activity. A few examples follow:

- **Drug use.** Your patient has reluctantly admitted to excessive alcohol use, and you strongly suspect abuse of illicit drugs. Symptom expectation may encourage a straightforward, honest response.

    What sorts of drugs do you usually use when you're drinking?

- **Suicidality.** Your patient is profoundly depressed and has expressed feelings of hopelessness. You suspect SI, but you sense that the patient may be too ashamed to admit it. Rather than gingerly asking, "Have you had any thoughts that you'd be better off dead?," you might decide to use symptom expectation.

    What kinds of ways to hurt yourself have you thought about?

Remember to use this technique only when you suspect that the patient has engaged in the behavior. For example, the question "What kinds of recreational drugs do you use?" may be appropriate when interviewing a young male admitted for a suicidal gesture while intoxicated, but wildly inappropriate for a 70-year-old woman being assessed for dementia.

SYMPTOM EXAGGERATION

Frequently, a patient minimizes the degree of his pathology, either to fool you or himself. Symptom exaggeration or amplification (Shea 1988), often used with symptom expectation, is helpful in clarifying the severity of symptoms. The technique involves suggesting a frequency of a problematic behavior that is higher than your expectation, so that the patient feels that his actual, lower frequency of the behavior will not be perceived by you as being "bad."

How much vodka do you drink each day? Two fifths? Three? More?

How many times do you binge and purge each day? Five times? Ten times?

How many suicide attempts have you had since your last hospitalization? Four? Five?

As is true for symptom expectation, you must reserve this technique for situations in which it seems appropriate. For example, if you have no reason to suspect that a patient has a drinking problem, asking how many cases of beer he drinks each day will sound quite insulting!

REDUCTION OF GUILT

While it is true that all the techniques in this chapter boil down to reducing a patient's sense of shame and guilt, the reduction-of-guilt technique seeks to directly reduce a patient's guilt about a specific behavior in order to discover what he has been doing. This technique is especially useful in obtaining a history of domestic violence and other antisocial behavior.

Domestic Violence

> I: *When you argue with your wife, does she ever throw things at you or hit you?*
>
> P: *She sure does. See this scar? She threw a vase at me 2 years ago.*
>
> I: *Do you fight back?*
>
> P: *Well, yes. I've bruised her a few times. Nothing compared to what she did to me.*

Another version of this technique is to begin by asking about other people:

> I: *Do you have any friends who push around their wives or girlfriends when they have an argument?*
>
> P: *Sure. They get pushed back, too.*
>
> I: *Have you done that yourself, pushed or hit your wife?*
>
> P: *Yeah. I'm not proud of it, but I've done it when she's gotten out of hand.*

Antisocial Behavior

> I: *Have you ever had any legal problems?*
>
> P: *Oh, here and there. A little shoplifting. Normal stuff.*

I: *Really? What was the best thing you ever stole?*

P: *The best thing? Well, I was into cars for a while. I spent a week cruising around in a Porsche 924, but I returned it. I was just into joyrides. Everyone was doing it back then.*

In this example, the interviewer used induction to bragging to reduce the patient's sense of guilt and lead to an admission of something more significant than shoplifting.

USE FAMILIAR LANGUAGE WHEN ASKING ABOUT BEHAVIORS

Sudman and Bradburn (1987) compared two methods of asking about alcohol use and sexuality. In the first method, they used "standard" language—words and phrases such as *intoxicated* and *sexual intercourse*. In the second method, they used "familiar," or "poetic" language—the language their respondents used for the same behavior, like *getting loaded* and *making love*. They found that the use of familiar language increased reports of these behaviors by 15%.

Apparently patients feel more comfortable admitting to socially undesirable behaviors if they feel the interviewer "speaks their language." The table below suggests various colloquial expressions to use in place of more formal language.

Using familiar language

Instead of:	Say:
Do you have a history of intravenous drug use?	Have you ever shot up?
Do you smoke marijuana?	Do you get high? Do you smoke dope?
Do you use cocaine?	Do you snort coke? Smoke crack?

5

Asking Questions II: Tricks for Improving Patient Recall

Essential Concepts

- Anchor questions to memorable events.
- Tag questions with specific examples.
- Describe syndromes in your patient's terms.

> Uttering a word is like striking a note on the keyboard of the imagination.
>
> Ludwig Wittgenstein

Throughout the diagnostic interview, your patient's memory will be both your ally and your enemy. Even when the desired information is not threatening in any way, be prepared for major inaccuracies and frustration if the events described occurred more than a few months ago. Nonetheless, we've all had the in-training experience of watching an excellent teacher elicit large quantities of historical information from a patient for whom we could barely determine age and sex. How do they do it? Here are some tricks of the trade.

ANCHOR QUESTIONS TO MEMORABLE EVENTS

Researchers have found that most people forget dates of events that occurred more than 10 days in the past (Azar 1997). Instead, we remember the distant past in relation to memorable events or periods (Sudman and Bradburn 1987), such as major transitions (graduations and birthdays), holidays, accidents or illnesses, major purchases (a house or a car), seasonal events ("the great blizzard of '78"), or public events (such as the O. J. Simpson trial or Princess Diana's death).

As an example, suppose you are interviewing a young woman with depression. You find out over the course of the interview that she has a heavy drinking history, and you want to determine which came first, the alcoholism or the depression. You could ask, "How many years ago did you begin drinking?" followed by "How many years ago did you become depressed?" but chances are you won't get an accurate answer to either question. Instead, use the anchoring technique:

> I: *Did you drink when you graduated from high school?*
>
> P: *I was drinking a lot back then, every weekend at least. Graduation week was one big party.*
>
> I: *Were you depressed then, too?*
>
> P: *I think so.*
>
> I: *How about when you first started high school? Were you drinking then?*
>
> P: *Oh no, I didn't really start drinking until I hooked up with my best friend toward the end of my freshman year.*
>
> I: *Were you depressed when you started school?*
>
> P: *Oh yeah, I could barely get up in time to make it to classes, I was so down.*

You've succeeded in establishing that her depression predated her alcoholism, which may have important implications for treatment.

TAG QUESTIONS WITH SPECIFIC EXAMPLES

In Chapter 8, you'll learn about the value of multiple-choice questions in limiting overly talkative patients. Tagging with examples is similar to posing multiple-choice questions, but it is used specifically for areas in which your patient is having trouble with recall. You simply tag a list of examples onto the end of your question.

To ascertain what medications your patient has taken in the past for depression, for example:

> I: *What were the names of the medications you took back then?*
>
> P: *Who knows? I really don't remember.*
>
> I: *Was it Prozac, Paxil, Zoloft, Elavil, Pamelor?*
>
> P: *Pamelor, I think. It gave me a really dry mouth.*

DEFINE TECHNICAL TERMS

Sometimes what appears to be a patient's vague recall is actually a lack of understanding of terms. For example, suppose you are interviewing a 40-year-old man with depression, and you want to determine when he had his first episode:

> I: *How old were you when you first remember feeling depressed?*
>
> P: *I don't know. I've always been depressed.*

You suspect that you and the patient have different meanings of depression, and you alter your approach:

> I: *Just to clarify: I'm not talking about the kind of sadness that we all experience from time to time. I'm trying to understand when you first felt what we call a clinical depression, and by that I mean that you were so down that it seriously affected your functioning, so that, for example, it might have interfered with your sleep, your appetite, and your ability to concentrate. When do you remember first experiencing something that severe?*
>
> P: *Oh, that just started a month ago.*

6 Asking Questions III: How to Change Topics with Style

Essential Concepts

- Use smooth transitions to cue off something the patient just said.
- Use referred transitions to cue off something said earlier in the interview.
- Use introduced transitions to pull a new topic from thin air.

Interviewing a patient for the first time requires touching on many different topics within a brief period. You'll need to constantly change the subject, which can be jarring and off-putting to a patient, especially when she is involved in an important and emotional topic. Skilled interviewers are able to change topics without alienating their patients and use various transitions to turn the interview into what Harry Stack Sullivan (1970) called a "collaborative inquiry."

SMOOTH TRANSITION

In the smooth transition (Sullivan 1970), you cue off something the patient just said in order to introduce a new topic. For example, a depressed patient is perseverating on conflicts with her husband and stepchildren; the interviewer wants to obtain information on family psychiatric history:

> P: *John has been good to me, but I can't stand the way his daughters expect me to go out of my way to make their lives easy; after all, they're adults!*
>
> I: *Speaking of family, has anyone else in your family been through the kind of depression that you've been going through?*

REFERRED TRANSITION

In the referred transition (Shea 1988), you refer to something the patient said earlier in the interview in order to move to a new topic. For example, at the beginning of an interview a depressed patient had briefly mentioned that he "didn't know if he could take this situation any more." Now, well into the evaluation, the interviewer wants to fully assess suicidality:

> P: *My doctor tried me on some medication for a while, but it didn't do much good.*

> I: *Earlier, you mentioned that you didn't know how much more of this you could take. Have you had the thought that you'd be better off dead?*

INTRODUCED TRANSITION

In the introduced transition, you introduce the next topic or series of topics before actually launching into it. This transition is often begun by a statement such as, "Now I'd like to switch gears . . ." or "I'd like to ask some different kinds of questions now." For example, you need to quickly run through the PROS, but you don't want the patient to feel that you are asking these questions because you expect that he actually suffers all these symptoms:

> I: *Now I'd like to switch gears a little and ask you about a bunch of different psychological symptoms that people sometimes have. Many of these may not apply to you at all, and that is a useful thing to know in itself.*

Techniques for the Reluctant Patient

7

Essential Concepts

- Use open-ended questions and commands to increase the flow of information.
- Use continuation techniques to keep the flow coming.
- Shift to neutral ground when necessary.
- Schedule a second interview when all else fails.

Occasionally, you run into the ideal patient. She's troubled and eager to talk. She briefly outlines the problems that led to her visit, and then answers each of your questions in full, stopping in preparation for your next query. You find that you've gathered all the vital information in 30 minutes, and you have the luxury of exploring her social and developmental history deeply. You feel like a real therapist. Your mind is whirring, and you can't wait to dust off that copy of Freud you bought the day you got into your training program but haven't had time to look at since.

Usually, however, your patient will fall somewhere on either side of a spectrum of information flow. Either he's not saying enough or he's saying too much, and it's not his fault. The average patient has no way of knowing what information is and is not important for a psychiatric diagnosis. It's up to you to educate the patient and to steer the interview appropriately.

OPEN-ENDED QUESTIONS AND COMMANDS

You can use open-ended questions and commands to increase the flow of information. Open-ended questions can't be answered with a simple "yes" or "no."

> *What kinds of symptoms has your depression caused?*

> *What sorts of things have you done when you felt manic?*

Open-ended commands are questions altered slightly to sound more directive.

Tell me what kinds of symptoms you've had.

Describe for me some of the things you've done while you were manic.

CLINICAL VIGNETTE

The patient was a woman in her 30s who had been admitted to the hospital after an overdose. She was unhappy with the involuntary admission and initially resistant to answering questions.

I: I understand that you took an overdose of your medicine last week.

P: Uh huh.

I: What do you think was going on? (An open-ended question.)

P: I don't know. (Which doesn't get anywhere.)

I: Were you feeling depressed?

P: Maybe.

I: Tell me a little about how you were feeling. (An open-ended command.)

P: There's not much to tell. I took the pills, that's all. (Still no results.)

I: I really want to help you, but the only way I can do that is to understand what was going through your head when you took the pills. (Some education, combined with another, more specific, command.)

P: I guess I thought it would be a good idea to take 'em. My husband was driving me crazy. (Now we're getting somewhere.)

CONTINUATION TECHNIQUES

Continuation techniques can be used to keep the flow coming. These expressions encourage a patient to continue revealing sensitive information:

- Go on.
- Uh huh.

- Continue with what you were saying about . . .
- Really?
- Wow.

They are often combined with facilitative body language, such as head nods, persistent eye contact, holding the chin between thumb and index finger, and facial emotional response to the material. Generally, the more spontaneous and genuine your responses to reluctant patients, the more likely you are to disarm them.

NEUTRAL GROUND

Some interviews begin badly and quickly deteriorate. For example, you may have had the experience of interviewing a patient who becomes increasingly alienated as your questions become more "psychiatric." If this happens, try changing the subject to something nonpsychiatric, with the intention of sidling back into your territory once you've gained the patient's trust.

I interviewed a college student who was referred by his dean for psychological evaluation after having said he would kill himself if he was not given a better grade in a course. He was an unwilling participant and had shown up only because he was threatened with suspension if he did not.

After the first 5 minutes of the interview, it was clear that he was not interested in talking about what was going through his mind, so I shifted to relatively neutral ground.

> I: *So how do you like college X?*
>
> P: *It's fine. There's a good English department.*
>
> I: *Really? Any particularly interesting classes?*
>
> P: *King Lear and the Modern World.*
>
> I: *It's been a while since I read that. How is King Lear related to the modern world?*
>
> P: *It's all about money and power. Everyone sucks up to King Lear because he has all this land to give away. It's the same way with lobbyists in Washington. Or professors at a university.*
>
> I: *Is that the way it is at your college?*
>
> P: *Of course. Professors sit in their offices, fat and happy, and students mean nothing to them. Unless they can get you to be their slave.*

This led to a discussion of his frustrations with school, which in turn led to his revealing the extent of his depressive symptoms.

SECOND INTERVIEW

When all else fails, you may need to schedule a second interview. If you're not getting anywhere with the patient, no matter how many interviewing tricks you use, you may need to cut the interview short with a comment such as

> *Why don't we stop for now and meet again next week [or tomorrow, for inpatient work]. That will give you a chance to think more about the sorts of things that are bothering you, and we can take it from there.*

I've done this several times, and the patient is usually more forthcoming at the next interview. I'm not sure why this works. Maybe giving the message that I accept their reluctance paradoxically encourages them to open up, or perhaps they feel awkward about not answering questions two interviews in a row.

Of course, before you end the interview, you must feel comfortable that the patient is not at imminent risk of suicide or other dangerous behaviors.

8

Techniques for the Overly Talkative Patient

Essential Concepts

- Use closed-ended and multiple-choice questions to limit the flow.
- Perfect the art of the gentle interruption.
- Educate the patient about the need to move along in the interview.

A man does not seek to see himself in running water, but in still water. For only what is itself still can impart stillness into others.

Chuang-tzu

It was the end of a long day in the crisis clinic, and I picked up the last chart. I ushered the patient, a middle-aged woman, into the interview room. She was well-groomed and socially appropriate, and she smiled warmly as she sat down. A good sign, I thought. She did not look like the sort of person who would need to be hospitalized, which is a time-consuming and exhausting process.

"How can I be of help today?" I asked.

"I am so glad I came here today," she responded. "I cannot tell you how terrible my life is. Sometimes I just don't think it's worthwhile going on. It began 21 years ago, when my first husband—a hard-drinking bastard, a real womanizer, someone I really should never have hooked up with and I wouldn't have if my parents hadn't nixed every other guy they met—and I can tell you, it was no picnic growing up in Westchester, because even though the average income is half a million, they treat their kids rotten."

A virtual torrent of information followed. For the next hour I struggled to rein in her circumstantial and wandering stories and to get at the kernel of her complaint.

The problem with overly talkative patients is how to limit the flow of information without seeming insensitive and impatient. Cox et al. (1988), in an experimental study of interviewing techniques, found the following techniques useful for "overly expressive patients":

- Closed-ended and multiple-choice questions
- Redirecting questions to another topic
- Structuring statements regarding information required and/or clinical procedures

In general, they found that a "brisk, highly controlling style" was helpful in limiting overly expressive patients, without alienating them.

USE CLOSED-ENDED AND MULTIPLE-CHOICE QUESTIONS

Although open-ended questions should be used with most patients, they will tend to increase the talkativeness of circumstantial patients. With such patients, the open-ended approach might result in something like the following:

> I: *How have you been sleeping?*
>
> P: *Not great. Who knows, though? Do you think I've been keeping track, with each one of my kids coming at me with a different problem, one kid a day, and with work calling to ask when I'm coming back, and . . .*

Closed-ended questions seek brief, "yes" or "no" replies or refer to a limited range of possible answers. Thus,

> *Have you been sleeping normally over the past week?*

is a closed-ended question, because it can be answered with a "yes" or "no." The following sleep question is also closed ended:

> *How many hours of sleep did you get last night?*

Although this one can't be answered with a "yes" or "no," it does refer to a limited number of possible responses, somewhere from "none" to "12 hours."

Multiple-choice questions limit answers to a greater extent than do closed-ended questions. They include a list of options for possible answers to the question, giving your patient guidance as to the level of precision expected. They are often useful in asking about the neurovegetative symptoms of depression:

> *How has your appetite been over the past few weeks: better than normal, worse than normal, or normal?*

> *What sort of sleep problem do you have? Problems*
> *falling asleep? Waking up throughout the night? Waking*
> *up too early in the morning?*

A common criticism of multiple-choice questions is that they may bias the patient toward one of your prepackaged answers. Cox et al. (1981b) examined this issue and found that patients were not biased in their replies, and that multiple-choice questions frequently yielded clear, on-topic answers.

Generally, you should sprinkle the interview with closed-ended and multiple-choice questions to rein in an overly talkative patient or with any patient with whom you have a lot of ground to cover in a very short time, such as in an emergency room evaluation. Be judicious in using these kinds of questions because some patients are alienated by them, and you risk turning a talkative patient into a terminally reluctant patient.

THE ART OF THE GENTLE INTERRUPTION

Although it may feel impolite to interrupt your patient, you're doing him no favor by letting him ramble for so long that you have insufficient time to do a proper evaluation. In some cases, you need to take charge of the interview actively. If you can accomplish this with sensitivity, you will not alienate your patient. In my experience, patients with a rambling, circumstantial style are so used to being interrupted that they barely flinch when you cut in; in fact, they often appear grateful, especially if they are working themselves into a state of anxiety or anger with their train of thought.

The gentle interruption is also known as a "redirecting statement" (Cox et al. 1988), and it comes in various guises.

In the **empathic interruption**, you add an empathic statement to soften the blow:

> *I can tell that this situation's been really hard for you*
> *to deal with. Have you been drinking lately, to cope*
> *with it?*

In the **delaying interruption**, you assure the patient that her topic is important and that you'd like to come back to it later:

> *I can see you feel strongly about your daughter's school*
> *troubles, and that's something we can talk about later,*
> *but right now I need to ask you about some of those*

> *signs of depression you were experiencing. Was your appetite normal through all this?*

Of course, there's also a note of empathy in that delaying statement.

The **educating interruption** incorporates a structuring statement in which you educate the patient about the sorts of questions you have yet to ask and the time constraints you're both working under. Usually this is done only after you've used the other two interruptions several times with no results.

> *I'm sorry, but I need to interrupt you again. We have about 20 minutes left and a lot of ground to cover, including your treatment history, your family background, and your medical history, and I want to make sure we have time at the end to talk about some medication changes. You can help by trying to answer the questions directly and not getting too sidetracked. How does that sound?*

or,

> *It's important that I learn more about how you've been eating and sleeping so that I can tell whether you're suffering from a clinical depression, so I may continue to interrupt you to get that important information.*

or, more simply,

> *We really have a lot of ground to cover over the next half hour, so I'm going to have to ask you a lot of questions. This may mean some interruptions, okay?*

Techniques for the Adolescent Patient*

Essential Concepts	
• Involve the family.	
• Overcome the "I don't know" syndrome.	
• Develop strategies for asking about drugs, sex, and conduct problems.	

Don't laugh at a youth for his affectations; he is only trying on one face after another to find his own.

Logan Pearsall Smith

There are three reasons to include a chapter on adolescents in a book otherwise devoted to adult psychopathology: (a) Child and adolescent treatment is a part of most general training programs; (b) many primarily "adult" clinicians are called on to evaluate adolescents; and (c) many "adult" patients are still struggling through late adolescence, which begins during the later teen years and extends to the early 20s. If you can master the techniques of evaluating adolescents, you will find yourself using these same techniques for many of your adult patients, of *any* age.

THE FAMILY INTERVIEW

Your initial interview with an adolescent will usually include family members for at least part of, and sometimes all of, the session. Adolescents are great minimizers and deniers, and you often will need to interview the family separately to ascertain the presence of any problem at all. In addition, many psychiatric disorders in adolescents are strongly related to family issues, with family dynamics sometimes contributing significantly to them (e.g., oppositional defiant disorder, depression) and at other times being the cause of family strife [e.g., attention-deficit hyperactivity disorder (ADHD)]. Finally,

*With contributions from David Sorenson, M.D., and Alan Lyman, M.D.

treatment can rarely happen without the consent and cooperation of family members.

Thus, for the first appointment, plan to invite the entire family into your office. Usually, I walk out to the waiting room and greet the patient with an introduction and handshake, then face the family, saying, "Why don't we all go in for the first part of the hour, then maybe I can have some time to chat with _____ afterward."

Once in the office, allow the family to decide where to sit, and then shut up and listen for a while, just as you would with your adult patients. If there is some initial silence, you can get things going with questions such as

> *What brings us all together today?*

> *What sort of issues have been coming up?*

or, more simply,

> *Okay, who wants to do the talking?*

A parent usually begins, and it is important that you listen closely, because a family's desires may be quite different from what you suspected or from what you can provide.

CLINICAL VIGNETTE

Two parents brought in their 17-year-old son for an evaluation. Once in the office, the mother's first words were, "I want you to commit my son for his drug addiction."

The son, taken aback, turned to her and said, "Are you crazy?"

What developed was that the parents had suspected the son of drug use, but had told him that this was a family therapy meeting to "work out some family issues." The mother's expectation was that the clinician would immediately have a police officer escort the patient from the office to a substance abuse treatment facility. The clinician explained that this was not possible, and went on to explain the state's legal criteria for involuntary commitment. Eventually, the adolescent agreed to outpatient treatment of substance abuse and depression.

Allow at least 5 minutes of free speech, in which you simply listen to family members discussing the perceived problem. Aside from clueing you into diagnostic possibilities, this will allow you to understand the communication style and family dynamics. After listening for a few minutes, you will want to jump in with various questions to ascertain elements of the psychiatric and social history. It is important to adopt a neutral attitude so as not to appear that you are taking the parents' side. If the parents constantly speak over the patient (or vice versa), make a corrective comment, such as

> Everyone obviously has a lot of feelings about this issue, but it is important that I get a chance to hear everyone's viewpoint without too much interrupting.

After a period of time, you will want to talk to the adolescent alone.

> I enjoyed meeting you, and now I'd like to talk about some things with Matthew. Afterwards we'll get back together and discuss what we've talked about.

THE INDIVIDUAL INTERVIEW

Initial Questions and Strategies

How much time should you devote to the individual interview? There are no hard-and-fast rules. A full hour of individual discussion may be appropriate for a sensitive and sophisticated 14-year-old adolescent with depression, whereas an angry and involuntary 17-year-old adolescent with conduct disorder may be able to tolerate no more than 5 minutes alone with you. The more verbal and engaged the patient seems, the more time you will want to allot for your individual interview with her.

So there you are, in the room alone with your adolescent patient. Clinicians who spend most of their time with adults often freeze at this point. What do you say to a 15-year-old, who may feel quite awkward and embarrassed, especially now that his parents have left the room?

You want to avoid awkward gaps in the conversation as much as possible, which may involve doing more talking than you normally do. Some degree of self-disclosure may be acceptable too, to build rapport. You can start with some tension-relieving statements such as

> Okay. Now I get to hear your side of the story.

> We have a half hour or so to talk confidentially now. I hope you'll feel comfortable telling me your side of what's been going on at home.

If the family discussion was heated, react to that in some way:

> *Whew, things got pretty hot there, what do you think?*

Remember that adolescents may have had no prior experience with a professional who asks very personal questions. Thus, it may be helpful to begin with a comment such as

> *Do you mind if I ask you some personal questions?*

> *I may ask some questions that you're uncomfortable answering, and you don't have to answer if you don't want to.*

At some point during the interview, say something about the limits of confidentiality. Relay the statement with terms such as "worry":

> *I won't tell your parents about anything you say unless I'm really worried that your life might be in danger.*

Later, before you bring the family back in, ask

> *Is there anything you don't want me to tell your parents?*

> *Is it okay if I tell your parents about these things?*

If they say "yes," follow up with

> *Do you want to tell them or do you want me to?*

This way, you're maximizing your patient's sense of control.

"I Don't Know" Syndrome

Adolescents tend to have difficulty describing their internal emotional state. Sometimes this is because they don't want to seem vulnerable; other times it's because their emotional vocabulary is underdeveloped. Thus, asking direct questions about feelings is likely to lead to the following type of exchange:

> I: *Have you been feeling depressed?*

> P: *I don't know.*

> I: *Have you been feeling angry?*

> P: *I don't know.*

> I: *How have you been feeling?*

> P: *Okay, I guess.*

How does one get beyond the "I don't know" syndrome? One way is to give the patient permission to plead the fifth:

> *Look, if you really don't know something, that's fine. But if you don't want to tell me something, that's OK too. Just say, "I don't want to say."*

Another strategy is to ask the "fly on the wall" question:

> *If I were a fly on the wall when you get into one of your moods, what would I see?*

or, a slight variation,

> *What would your friend look like if he looked like you in one of your moods?*

These questions invite the patient to describe his behavior, a less threatening proposition than describing a subjective state.

A third strategy is to rely on the defense mechanism of displacement. Ask your patient if he has any friends with problems:

> *Do you have any friends who are in trouble? What's going on with them?*

This might lead into an elaborate discussion of a friend's antisocial or suicidal behavior, which may actually be *auto*-biographical.

Topics to Cover

Often the trick with adolescents is to get them talking, much less getting them to reveal personal information. The best strategy is to adopt an attitude of curiosity and respect; a sense of humor is always a plus.

Most adolescents are interested in music, so this is as good a place to start as any.

> *Do you like music? Who do you like?*

Chances are that you will have never heard of their favorite group. You could respond with

> *I have no idea what kind of music that is. Me, I like jazz and, I'm ashamed to admit, Barry Manilow.*

If you're square and goofy, and most of us over 30 are, admit it. This is disarming to most adolescents and is better than trying to pose as "cool."

Asking about School and Other Activities

Other questions that help open up a shut-down adolescent include questions about school, friends, and interests. Each line of inquiry can also serve as a jumping-off point for diagnostic questions.

> *Where do you go to school?*
>
> *What's that school like?*
>
> *Is it fun?*
>
> *Is it easy?*
>
> *What are the other kids like there?*
>
> *Who do you hang out with?*

After asking these nonthreatening questions, ask about grades. If his grades are low or if he looks disappointed in his grades, follow up with

> *Is that the same as you've always done, or have your grades changed recently?*

A change in grades may signal the onset of depression or involvement with substance abuse. You might also ask

> *Are there any particular subjects that are hard?*

The *DSM-IV* classifies learning disorders under the traditional categories of reading, writing, and arithmetic, and you can pick up a hint of a learning disorder by asking this question. However, children are usually diagnosed with a learning disability long before their teenage years.

> *What do you do with your time after school?*

Are you involved in any extracurricular activities, like sports or clubs?

> *What do you enjoy doing the most?*

Besides being good questions for opening up your patient and establishing rapport, these are good screening questions for depression. Withdrawal from social activities is a common feature of teenage depression. Conversely, the patient who expresses clear interest and excitement in *any* activity is less likely to be depressed.

> *How many hours of TV do you watch on the average school night?*

How many hours do you spend on the computer?

This gives another indication of how socially involved your patient is.

Asking about Drugs and Alcohol

Using the techniques discussed in Chapter 4 is helpful in communicating a nonjudgmental attitude when asking about drug use. Thus, you can use normalization:

> *I hear there's a lot of drinking and drug use at your school. Do you know anyone who uses drugs?*

> *You read in the paper that 90% of kids use drugs these days. Do you ever use drugs?*

or symptom expectation:

> *How often do you have a drink?*

> *What drugs do you use?*

Other patients respond quite well to a direct query:

> *Do you drink or use drugs?*

Asking about Sex

Although asking about sex is important when interviewing adolescents, use judgment and common sense in determining when such questions are appropriate. If your rapport is shaky, you may want to delay such questions for follow-up visits, or you may decide not to raise the questions at all. It's vitally important that any questions about sex *not* be seen by your patient as idle or lurid interest, but rather that they are seen as an essential component of your psychiatric evaluation. A sexual history is important for a variety of psychiatric and medical issues, including assessing risk for AIDS; discovering a history of sexual abuse; and assessing the presence of sexual acting-out as a symptom of depression, mania, substance abuse, or other disorder.

A good way to approach this uncomfortable topic is to begin talking about "romance" rather than "sex."

> *Do you have any romantic relationships?*

> *How long have you been seeing this person?*

> *What's his/her name?*

> *What do you like about _____?*

Now that you've given a human face to the relationship, you can introduce the topic of sex:

> *Would you feel comfortable if we talked about your sex life?*
>
> *Are you sexually active?*
>
> *Are you using protection?*
>
> *Do you know about AIDS?*
>
> *Do you ever do things sexually that you later regret, like not using protection or having sex with people you don't know very well?*

You can also approach sexuality by embedding it in a list of health-related questions:

> *I want to ask a few questions about your health:*
>
> *Do you get headaches?*
>
> *Stomachaches?*
>
> *Do you have sexual problems?*
>
> *Are you sexually active?*
>
> *Do you smoke?*
>
> *Do you use drugs or alcohol?*

If it seems appropriate, ask about sexual orientation:

> *Have you ever wondered whether your sexual feelings are normal?*
>
> *Do you ever think that your feelings about sex are different from other kids' feelings?*

Note that neither of these questions uses terms such as *sexual orientation* and *sexual identity*, either of which may confuse or alienate adolescents.

Asking about Conduct Problems

Conduct disorder and oppositional defiant disorder are common reasons for referral, and you'll often be faced with the task of getting patients to admit to illegal behavior. Usually, the parents will have disclosed such behavior during the family meeting. A good way to begin a private interview in such circumstances is as follows:

> *It looks like your mom feels there's been a lot of stealing (or whatever alleged behavior) and I have no way of knowing if it's true, but if you were stealing, I'm sure there was a good reason for it. Maybe it was the only way you could get something? Or maybe your friends challenged you to do it?*

or, more simply,

> *Do you know what your parents are saying about what you've been doing?*

If the rapport is good, and you don't mind using some humor, use the "inducing to brag" approach:

> *So, I hear you're an excellent thief. What's the best thing you've stolen?*

Remember that you aren't asking these questions just to get your patient to confess to bad behaviors; rather, you're primarily interested in finding out why he does these things. Is it peer pressure? A way of expressing anger toward his parents? A symptom of a manic episode? Follow up on an admission of antisocial behaviors with questions designed to address these topics.

10 ▼ Techniques for Other Challenging Situations

> **Essential Concepts**
> - The Hostile Patient
> - The Seductive Patient
> - The Tearful Patient

Be firm, fair, and understanding. Hold the reins in one hand and a lump of sugar in the other.

Elvin Semrad
The Heart of a Therapist

THE HOSTILE PATIENT

When a patient becomes hostile during an initial interview, remember that it's not your fault. Unless you're laughably incompetent or a real creep, a hostile attack is a product of the patient's pathology. Common causes of patient anger during the first meeting include paranoid psychosis, irritability due to depression or mania, and borderline personality disorder. The best way to defuse hostility is to diagnose its cause and then target your intervention accordingly.

The Hostile, Paranoid Patient

The hostile, paranoid patient is angry at you because he perceives you as a direct threat or perhaps as part of an elaborate conspiracy. A good way to counteract this false projection is to use self-effacing humor or general goofiness, which is easier to pull off. The patient usually perceives this attitude as inconsistent with evil intentions.

CLINICAL VIGNETTE

A patient with the diagnosis of bipolar disorder was admitted involuntarily to the inpatient unit because of paranoia concerning her husband, who she believed was trying to have her killed. It was clear from the outset of the interview that she felt that she had been wrongly committed and wanted to leave immediately.

> P: *How can you keep me here? You have no right. I can call a lawyer.*
>
> I: *You can certainly call a lawyer. The reason we . . .*
>
> P: *(Interrupting) I can call a lawyer, but it's not going to do any good, is it? All the lawyers are part of a big game and they're going to say just what you want them to say.*
>
> I: *What kind of game do you think this is? Last I checked, this was just a psychiatric hospital.*
>
> P: *You know exactly what's going on here, and wipe that innocent look off your face.*
>
> I: *I'm not innocent. I plead guilty to being a psychiatrist. I'm trying to help you. And if you believe that, I have a bridge in Brooklyn you might be interested in.*
>
> P: *What bridge?*
>
> I: *Oh that's just an old joke, and a bad one. I find that I have to use humor to keep me sane here, you know? But enough about me. What were we talking about?*
>
> P: *The people who are trying to have me killed.*

At this point, the patient opened up significantly, and a productive conversation ensued. The attempt at humor was unexpected enough to derail an increasingly hostile train of thought.

The Irritable, Depressed Patient

Depressed patients can come across as hostile, but it is a hostility that cloaks a reservoir of pain. A good technique is to make a fairly direct interpretation, such as

> *You sound angry, but I think there's some sadness underneath that anger.*
>
> *I can understand how you would be angry with me, but I wonder if there isn't something beneath the anger that's eating at you?*

The Patient with Borderline Personality Disorder

Like the irritable, depressed patient, the borderline patient's anger overlies pain. Because of immature coping skills, the patient cannot "sit" with her pain and rationally problem-solve. Instead, she tends to project and externalize, resulting in lashing out that can be quite uncomfortable for you. It isn't easy to maintain your composure during these times, but it helps if you can see the anger as a crisis of aloneness. Be compassionate, and fight against the natural tendency to either fight back or to withdraw into a protective shell of aloofness. Defensiveness will only rile your patient further, and aloofness will deepen her sense of abandonment.

Instead, be curious, interested, and caring. Effective statements for patients with borderline personality disorder often include the following:

> *For the sake of our discussion, what do you think just happened? You're very angry at me, and I'm wondering what that anger is about.*

> *I've done (or said) something that upset you, and I hope to understand what that is so that we can put it behind us and move on with the important work we have to do to help you feel better.*

THE SEDUCTIVE PATIENT

While seductive behavior often does not become apparent until follow-up sessions, it is helpful to have some idea of how best to respond to overtly seductive behavior. To begin with, renew your own absolute commitment never to become sexually involved with your patients. Aside from breaking professional ethical codes, it is always destructive, to both your patient and yourself. Any practitioner who often finds himself tempted to breach this boundary should get therapy or supervision or find another career.

This is not to say that you will never have sexual feelings toward your patients. Of course you will, but if your commitment never to act on such feelings is absolute, you can manage these feelings while continuing to deliver excellent care.

Seductive behavior comes in two guises, subtle and blatant. Subtle behavior includes significant glances, revealing clothes, and excessive curiosity about the interviewer's personal life. Such subtle behavior can be managed in several ways:

- Keep the trappings of the therapeutic relationship relatively formal.
- Use the patient's title and last name.
- Keep the interview focused on the presenting symptoms.
- Avoid small talk.

Deflect requests for personal information with statements such as "The purpose of this interview is for us to get a better understanding of what's been troubling you, and I really think that should be the focus."

Blatant seductive behavior involves more direct questions about the interviewer's availability and requests to be touched or hugged by the therapist or to spend some time outside of the treatment session with her. These behaviors require a direct and unambiguous response that makes it clear such contact is inappropriate and impossible and explains why. The following vignette illustrates this type of situation.

CLINICAL VIGNETTE

The patient is a woman in her 30s who is in the process of divorcing her husband. She has scheduled a diagnostic interview to evaluate her depression. The interviewer is a married man also in his 30s. The vignette begins toward the end of the interview, and the clinician has already recommended an antidepressant.

I: *I also think it would be helpful for you to see a therapist.*

P: *Can't you be my therapist?*

I: *No, I'm a psychopharmacologist, and I schedule brief follow-up visits to check on how well the medication is working.*

P: *But I like you.*

I: *(Beginning to sense a hint of seductiveness.) That's good, because I'll continue to monitor your medication, but I think you'd benefit from seeing a therapist for more frequent sessions.*

P: *(Smiling seductively.) What I'd really like is to meet someone who could be both my therapist and my lover.*

> I: *Wait a minute. Let's back up a little. It's very destructive for therapists or psychiatrists to have anything other than a professional relationship with their patients. That will never happen during our treatment, nor will it happen with any therapist you might see. From what you've told me today, I can see you've been feeling lonely, and I think it would be good for you to work on building up friendships, but that will have to happen outside of treatment sessions.*

The patient eventually accepted a therapy referral and continued in treatment without overt seductiveness.

THE TEARFUL PATIENT

Many patients cry during the initial appointment, and as a beginning clinician you may feel at a loss when this happens. You will typically feel your own share of emotions in such situations, which may range from poignant empathy to anxious discomfort. You will probably instinctively want to behave as you would when a close friend or family member cries in front of you, which may include a pat or a hug and comforting words. That is usually a mistake in a professional relationship. So what should you do?

The proper approach will vary from patient to patient. When a patient cries, try to understand the meaning of the tears, which is not always obvious. For example, the patient who cries while describing a recent marital separation may be crying for several reasons, including a feeling of abandonment, a fear of future financial hardship, a sense of personal failure, and a relief that the relationship is over.

When a patient becomes tearful, I recommend offering some tissues, which should always be in your office, waiting empathetically for a few seconds, and then asking any of the following questions:

> *What is it about what you are saying that is so painful?*
>
> *I can see you're feeling emotional now; what are your tears about?*
>
> *What's on your mind now as you're crying?*

It's also helpful to ask about the frequency of crying:

> *Have you been crying a lot about this?*

It's quite common for patients to say they have not cried until that very moment, which is usually a validation of your interviewing skills.

If a patient expresses some shame or embarrassment about crying, make a validating statement such as

> *Crying can be a good release.*

> *Go ahead and cry as much as you need to. It's good that you feel comfortable enough here that you're allowing yourself to cry.*

> *Crying is a big part of the healing process.*

Of course, lest I leave you with the impression that crying is a wonderful thing, I should remind you that tears indicate intense emotional pain and should prompt you to be especially vigilant for suicidal ideation (see Chapter 20).

Practical Psychodynamics in the Diagnostic Interview

Essential Concepts
- Assess your patient's degree of reality distortion.
- Detect negative transference and move beyond it.
- Identify defense mechanisms and coping responses.
- Use your countertransference diagnostically.

It might be said of psychoanalysis that if you give it your little finger it will soon have your whole hand.

Sigmund Freud

Keeping an ear open for psychodynamic material can help you in a number of ways as you conduct your diagnostic interviews. First, you can increase the accuracy of your diagnosis, since symptoms are often the product of life circumstances and dysfunctional ways of responding to them. Psychodynamics provides the preeminent language for describing **defense mechanisms**, and it also helps you understand how to use countertransference toward patients productively. Second, understanding psychodynamic principles will help you manage the interview itself, especially if your patient has negative transference towards you. Finally, understanding defense mechanisms will help you to diagnose personality disorders, which are covered in more detail in Chapter 28.

REALITY DISTORTION

Reality distortion is often the first clue that significant psychodynamic factors may be at work in your patient's psychology. Psychosis is the extreme of reality distortion, but many nonpsychotic patients distort reality as well. Examples include the depressed woman who unfairly castigates herself for being the cause of all misfortune in her family, the narcissist who tells you that all his past therapists have been substandard and therefore unhelpful, and the alcoholic who says her husband is being ridiculous in criticizing her drinking habits.

Often, reality distortions will jump out at you over the course of the interview. Occasionally, you'll need to dig for them. In Chapter 25, I suggest some screening questions to elicit the presence of the delusions. In these patients, however, we're not talking about frank delusions; we're talking about milder distortions. The way to elicit distortions is to be curious about how your patient interprets the motivations of others or how they make sense of events overall.

CLINICAL VIGNETTE

The patient is a 25-year-old woman with a history of panic disorder with agoraphobia and comorbid alcohol abuse. She recently terminated visits to her last psychiatrist because he refused to prescribe benzodiazepines for her anxiety disorder.

> P: *Dr. X said, "Absolutely not. I won't give you any Xanax."*
>
> I: *What do you think was on his mind when he said that? (You are probing for her world view.)*
>
> P: *To tell you the truth, I have no idea. Maybe that's his rule.*
>
> I: *What sort of rule do you mean?*
>
> P: *Maybe he never prescribes those kinds of drugs for people like me.*
>
> I: *People like you?*
>
> P: *People with anxiety, people who really need them.*
>
> I: *Why wouldn't he prescribe meds to people who need them?*
>
> P: *Who knows. He's probably burned out. Most shrinks are.*

The patient presents a jaded view of psychiatrists, possibly reflecting a more general view of the world as uncaring. Alternatively, her statements may reflect the defense mechanism of projection, in which the patient disavows her own anger at being deprived of an addictive drug and projects it onto her psychiatrist, who then appears sadistic to her because he doesn't prescribe medications to people who need them. Whatever the nature of her distortions, you can be certain that you will not be exempt from them, and you can begin to prepare your own strategy to prevent future struggles. This might include making statements that demonstrate an understanding of her world view:

> *As I listen to you, it sounds like you've gotten the short end of the stick over and over again in life. I wouldn't be surprised if you're assuming that it's going to be the same way here, too.*

Once you detect a reality distortion, determine whether defense mechanisms or transference is at work.

NEGATIVE TRANSFERENCE

> Whenever two people meet there are really six people present. There is each man as he sees himself, each man as the other person sees him, and each man as he really is.
>
> William James

In transference, your patient unconsciously reenacts a past relationship and transfers it to a present relationship; this doesn't necessarily pose a problem in the initial interview. Your patient may have a positive transference toward you, in which you remind him of someone he admired, like his mother, causing him to automatically ascribe to you all kinds of wonderful qualities. Sit back and enjoy it.

Negative transference, however, can be problematic, especially when it involves anger. Your patient may have been poorly treated by people throughout his life, and he expects you to be no different. Look for negative transference when there is a sense of tension. Perhaps your patient is making angry comments or asking provocative questions. Perhaps he is giving monosyllabic answers to your questions.

In psychoanalytic psychotherapy, negative transference is actually elicited, because its interpretation is the backbone of treatment. In the diagnostic interview, however, negative transference is usually counterproductive, and the best way to deal with it is to recognize it and make an empathic comment that neutralizes it. Although there's no easy way of learning how to make these comments—other than practice, practice, and more practice—the following list contains some common statements (in italics) made by patients during diagnostic interviews. Most of these statements reflect negative transference or a defense mechanism of some sort. All of these statements tend to throw novice interviewers for a loop.

Possible hidden meanings are listed after each patient statement; the emphasis is on *possible*. Sometimes, such statements have no hidden meaning and are a statement of fact. For example, you may look bored during an interview and, in fact, *feel* bored. If the patient is making an accurate observation, don't try to interpret the comment. That is dishonest and unfair to your patient. In addition, the hidden meanings I've listed are illustrative only. They don't imply that all patients making such a statement actually mean what I suggest. You should interpret each statement individually, based on your knowledge of the particular patient.

In general, the possible responses are ways of moving beyond the negative statement, so that the work of the diagnostic interview can proceed. Note that this is a very different approach from what you would do if you were engaged in psychodynamic therapy.

You're not a very helpful doctor.

Possible hidden meaning: No one has ever cared for me, and you're no exception.
Possible response (while nodding empathically): "You know, that's not the first time I've heard that, and when I'm not being helpful to a patient I always ask, 'How can I be more helpful? Because I really do want to help.'" (This communicates that you really do care, and implies that the therapeutic alliance won't be damaged by your patient's comment, but may actually be strengthened by it.)

Possible hidden meaning: I'm a very special patient, and you should treat me unusually well.
Possible response: "I bet it feels disappointing to have a doctor who doesn't come up to snuff. Is it possible, though, that you're judging prematurely?" (Empathize with the patient's injured sense of specialness, while giving him an out to repair the relationship.)

You look bored.

Possible hidden meaning: Of course you are bored, I'm such a boring person.

Possible response: "I'm actually not at all bored, but do you think that the things you're saying are boring?"

Possible hidden meaning: I expect you to respond lovingly and immediately to everything I say; if you are silent, I have to assume that you're feeling something negative toward me.
Possible response: "In my profession, silence rarely means boredom. It usually means concentration and interest."

> *Is that all you're going to do, just sit there silently and nod?*

Possible hidden meaning: You're just like my parents, who never expressed any kind of interest in me, who never responded to anything I said.
Possible response: "Does that seem unhelpful? I actually have a lot to say, but I always try to bite my tongue so that my patients get a chance to tell their whole story. I usually find that I'm most helpful to patients only after I've really listened to them and understood them well."

> *What kind of credentials do you have?*

Possible hidden meaning: I'm in a lot of pain, and I'm not certain whether you or anybody else can help me.
Possible response: (Begin by stating your credentials quickly.) "I'm _____ (e.g., an intern, a resident) at _____ (i.e., name of school or hospital). Are you concerned about my ability to help you?"

Possible hidden meaning: I've been made to feel ineffectual all my life, and I want you to get a taste of what that feels like. (This is an example of an immature defense mechanism known as *projective identification*.)
Possible response: (State your credentials.) "But my main credential is that I'm here with you; I want to understand you and to help you as best I can." (By this you demonstrate that self-esteem does not depend on getting someone else to say you are effectual.)

> *You don't show much understanding of what I'm saying.*

Possible hidden meaning: I'm angry at you for not understanding me implicitly and fully without my having to be explicit. I want you to be the perfectly empathic parent I never had.
Possible response: "You know, I couldn't agree more. It is so hard for one person to really understand another person. But why don't we talk some more, and I'll give it my best shot."

Are you married?

Possible hidden meaning: I wish I were married to you.
Another possible hidden meaning: I'll bet you are married, and that you have a wonderful spouse, proving how much better you are than I am and what a loser I am.
Possible response (with a smile): "Wait a minute! I thought *I* was the one who's supposed to be asking the questions here."
Another possible response: "You know what? I've found that when I start answering questions about my personal life, it can get in the way of my understanding you better, and isn't that the whole point of our hour together?"

DEFENSE MECHANISMS AND COPING RESPONSES

When uncomfortable and unpleasant emotions arise, we all have ways of lessening the brunt of them. We use defense mechanisms. The following classifications are adapted from Vaillant's (1988) hierarchy of defense mechanisms:

Classification of defense mechanisms

Mature defenses	Suppression
	Altruism
	Sublimation
	Humor
Neurotic defenses	Denial
	Repression
	Reaction formation
	Displacement
	Rationalization
Immature defenses	Passive aggression
	Acting out
	Dissociation
	Projection
	Splitting (idealization/devaluation)
Psychotic defenses	Denial of external reality
	Distortion of external reality

Adapted from Valliant, G. E. (1998). Defense mechanisms. In A. M. Nicholi, Jr. (Ed.), *The New Harvard Guide to Psychiatry*. Cambridge, MA: Harvard University Press, 81.

Main Defense Mechanisms

Following are brief definitions and examples of the different defense mechanisms. The examples included here are various ways that a patient might react if, in this instance, her husband left her.

Mature Defenses. Mature defenses usually arise from, and lead to, psychological health rather than from dysfunction.

SUPPRESSION
- Definition: Emotion remains conscious but is suppressed.
- Example: I'm disappointed and sad, but I won't let these emotions interfere significantly with my life.

ALTRUISM
- Definition: Suppressing the emotion by doing something nice for others.
- Example: I'll volunteer at a women's shelter.

SUBLIMATION
- Definition: Transmuting the emotion into a productive and socially redeeming endeavor.
- Example: I'll start immediately on a book about how to cope with rejection.

HUMOR
- Definition: Expressing the emotion in an indirect and humorous way.
- Example: This is great! I've been trying for years to get rid of 180 pounds of ugly fat.

Neurotic (Transitional) Defenses

Neurotic defenses are less healthy than mature defenses because they tend to cause psychological distress either immediately, as with repression or displacement, or in the future, when the actual pain eventually surfaces.

DENIAL
- Definition: Denying that the emotion exists.
- Example: The rejection doesn't bother me at all.

REPRESSION
- Definition: Stuffing the emotion out of conscious awareness. (Unfortunately, the emotion typically returns to haunt the repressor in unpredictable ways.)
- Example: I didn't feel at all bad about his leaving me, but for the past few weeks I've had this splitting headache, and I don't know why.

REACTION FORMATION
- Definition: Forgetting the negative emotion by transforming it into its opposite.
- Example: We've become such close friends since this happened. He is really a wonderful person.

DISPLACEMENT
- Definition: Displacing the emotion from its original object to something or someone else.
- Example: My boss has really been getting under my skin lately.

RATIONALIZATION
- Definition: Inventing a convincing, but usually false, reason why you are *not* bothered.
- Example: I've been wanting to make some major life changes anyway. This finally gave me the boost I needed to do all the things I've been wanting to do.

Immature Defenses
Immature defenses lead to more severe distress and often have a negative impact on other people.

PASSIVE AGGRESSION
- Definition: Expressing anger indirectly and passively.
- Example: Oh, I'm sorry, dear. I gave all your clothes to the Salvation Army last week. I didn't realize you wanted them.

ACTING OUT
- Definition: Expressing the emotion in action rather than keeping it in awareness.
- Example: (The patient makes harassing, late-night phone calls.)

DISSOCIATION
- Definition: Dissociating instead of feeling the pain.
- Example: I was really spaced out all of last week; my memory of him leaving me is very hazy.

PROJECTION
- Definition: Disavowing the anger and ascribing it to the object of the anger.
- Example: I'm convinced that ever since he left me he's been bad-mouthing me to all our friends.

SPLITTING (IDEALIZATION/DEVALUATION)
- Definition: Defining the rejecting person as being all bad, versus having seen him as all good before the rejection, thereby transforming pain into anger and accusation.

- Example: I always knew he was a horrible person, and this proves it. May he rot in hell.

Psychotic Defenses

Psychotic defenses so completely flaunt external reality that they signal a psychotic thought process (TP).

DENIAL OF EXTERNAL REALITY

- Definition is self-explanatory.
- Example: He never left me.

DISTORTION OF EXTERNAL REALITY

- Definition is self-explanatory.
- Example: He didn't leave me! He went off on a business trip. He'll be back next week.

In the diagnostic interview, identifying defense mechanisms is useful to quickly sense whether your patient may have a personality disorder (such patients typically use immature defenses) and to give you a sense of prognosis (patients who use higher level defenses tend to do better than others).

As you listen to your patient with a psychodynamic ear, ask yourself the following questions:

- How does the patient seem to shelter himself from the psychological pain that he is sharing with you?
- Does he tend to use mature or immature defenses?
- Do his defenses tend to bring him out of his misery (mature defenses) or steep him more deeply in it (neurotic and immature defenses)?
- If you were his therapist, which of his defenses would you encourage and which would you point out to him as unproductive?

At the end of the interview, before you write up the evaluation, you'll find it helpful to review the defenses (see the pocket cards in Appendix A) and determine which one(s) the patient seems to use. Make a habit of spending at least a few moments thinking about the defenses your patients use. This will help you to better recognize defenses in the future.

Coping Styles

Coping styles and defense mechanisms are similar concepts. Vaillant distinguishes coping responses from defense mechanisms: Coping, he says, "involves eliciting help from appropriate others" and "voluntary cognitive efforts like information gathering, anticipating danger, and rehearsing responses to danger" (Vaillant 1988, p. 200). Defense mechanisms, on the other hand, are *involuntary* cognitive responses to stressors that usually fit into one of the categories listed in the prior section.

Think of coping as a series of active behavioral and cognitive responses designed to overcome a stressful event. You will typically be able to evaluate your patient's coping styles by listening to her HPI and hearing how she dealt with the distress. It is not surprising that the coping responses of many psychiatric patients are not very effective.

How did your patient respond to the main problems described in the HPI? If depression is the problem, did he cope adaptively, by (for example) contacting friends or family for support; decreasing his responsibilities for a while; or doing something that he knew would give him pleasure, such as seeing a movie or going on a vacation? Or did he cope maladaptively, by isolating himself, by lashing out at people close to him, or through self-mutilating behavior?

If anxiety is a major problem, did he use positive coping strategies, such as telling himself the anxiety will pass, taking deep breaths, taking a walk? Or did he use more negative strategies, such as visiting hospital emergency rooms excessively, using alcohol or other drugs, or bingeing on sweets?

As with defense mechanisms, seek to encourage positive coping responses and to discourage negative ones.

USING COUNTERTRANSFERENCE DIAGNOSTICALLY

Countertransference refers to the whole range of emotions that you may feel toward your patient, whether positive or negative. Novice interviewers have a tendency to try to suppress or ignore such feelings, especially when they are negative. **Don't.** These countertransference feelings represent some of the most clinically valuable material available to you. Whatever feelings your patient elicits in you are feelings she probably elicits in most other people she encounters in her life. Knowing this can give you powerful insight into the nature of her problems.

CLINICAL VIGNETTE

A 45-year-old man was admitted to the psychiatric unit for depression and SI. He had recently been fired from his job, and he complained of loneliness, as he had lost most of his friends over the years. I did the admission interview, and the following exchange occurred 5 minutes into it.

> I: *How long had you been feeling depressed?*

> P: *Quite a while. But tell me, aren't you just a resident?*

> I: *(Immediately feeling defensive.) Well, yes, I'm the chief resident of the unit.*

> P: *(He narrows his eyes.) Chief resident. I see. That's a pretty political position, isn't it?*

> I: *(Increasingly uncomfortable and caught off guard.) No, I wouldn't say it's a particularly political position. I supervise the other residents.*

> P: *Yes, but there's always someone watching over you, isn't there? If you do well, maybe you'll get a nice job in the department. I know how it works. I'd prefer to talk to a full attending, someone who isn't always looking over his shoulder.*

> I: *(Feeling enraged and suppressing the urge to scream at him and kick him out of the office.) In fact, you will be talking to an attending in the morning, but I do need to talk to you briefly this afternoon.*

The patient agreed to proceed with the interview, and answered questions briefly and disdainfully. On further assessment, a picture of severe narcissistic personality disorder emerged, and my countertransference reaction made it graphically understandable how he had managed to alienate all the important people in his life, leading to his current depression.

The bottom line is that when you feel a negative emotion toward your patient, don't act on it. Instead, analyze its possible connection to your patient's psychopathology.

THE PSYCHIATRIC HISTORY

The unexamined life is not worth living.

Socrates

12 Obtaining the History of Present Illness

Essential Questions

- What has been happening over the past week or two that has brought you into the clinic?
- Have there been any events that you think have caused your problem or made it worse?
- Have you sought any treatment for this problem?

Recommended time: 10 minutes

WHAT IS THE HISTORY OF PRESENT ILLNESS?

HPI is probably the most important part of the psychiatric interview, and yet there is disagreement on exactly what it should entail. Even experienced clinicians differ in how they approach the HPI. Some think of it as the "history of present crisis" and focus on the preceding few weeks. Such clinicians begin their interviews with questions such as, "What has been going on recently that brings you into the clinic today?" Others begin by eliciting the entire history of the patient's primary syndrome: "Tell me about your depression. How old were you when you first felt depressed?" These clinicians work forward to the present episode.

Each of these approaches may be useful, depending on the clinical situation. If a patient has a relatively uncomplicated and brief psychiatric history, it might make sense to explore that first and then move to the HPI. If the psychiatric history is long, with many hospitalizations and caregivers, starting at the beginning may bring you too far from the present problem.

The most common pitfall for beginners is spending too much time on the HPI. It's easy to do, because this is the time for your patient to share the most difficult and painful part of his story, and cutting your patient off as time begins to pass may seem unempathic. Thus, it is vital that you keep in mind the advice offered in Part I about asking questions and changing topics sensitively. Use these techniques to gently but persistently bring the patient back to the HPI.

In the following sections, I describe techniques for the two major approaches to the HPI; you should decide which to use for a given patient.

The History of Present Crisis Approach

The *American Heritage Dictionary* defines *crisis* as "A crucial point or situation in the course of anything; a turning point." As you begin the interview, ask yourself, "Why now? Why is this a crucial point in this person's life? What has been happening recently to bring her into my office?" Often, psychiatric crises occur over a 1- to 4-week period, so focus your initial questions on this period.

> *What has been happening over the past week or two that has brought you into the clinic?*

> *Tell me about some of the stressors you've dealt with over the past couple of weeks.*

History of the Syndrome Approach

Alternatively, you can begin your questioning by ascertaining when the patient first remembers signs of the illness.

> *When did you first begin having these kinds of problems?*

> *When was the last time you remember feeling perfectly well?*

Ensuing questions track the course of the illness through months or years, arriving eventually at the present.

> *Now let's talk about this current episode. When did it start?*

One nice thing about this approach to the HPI is that most case write-ups are organized in this format—they often begin, "The patient was without any psychiatric problems until age 18, when she became depressed . . ."

ELICIT A CHRONOLOGIC NARRATIVE, EMPHASIZING PRECIPITANTS

Many patients automatically jump into a chronologic narrative of their problems when prompted by one of the preceding questions. If this happens, it is a time to fall silent for a while and listen. Remember, this is your "scouting period" (see

Chapter 3), during which you are observing, listening, and hypothesizing. However, if your patient begins to jump around into other issues or time frames, you may want to refocus him.

> P: *I felt so angry when my wife yelled at me. But she's always been that way. Back when I was in law school, she nagged at me constantly. I'd have to spend late nights at the law library, and she refused to understand.*

> I: *I'd like to hear more about that period later, but right now let's focus on what's been happening over the last 2 weeks or so. You said you got angry at her. What happened then?*

Ask the patient specifically about potential precipitants for her suffering:

> *Have there been any events that have caused your problem or made it worse?*

Occasionally, the patient will deny any precipitants. This is particularly true of patients who view their psychiatric illness from a medical model. Such a patient might answer the question above with

> *No, I can't think of anything that's causing it. My life is going pretty well; I just keep getting these depressions.*

Certainly, some psychiatric illnesses, such as bipolar disorder, can have lives of their own, but it's unusual for patients to decompensate without some precipitant. Often, patients haven't associated particular events with their pain and simply need their memories jogged. Make it a practice to dig by asking about specific events that commonly destabilize patients.

Common precipitants of psychiatric syndromes

Arguments with friends or relatives
Rejection or abandonment
Death or major illness of loved one
Anniversary of a negative event, such as a death or divorce
Major medical illness or age-related deterioration in functioning
Stressful events at work or school
Mental health clinician going on vacation
Medication noncompliance
Substance abuse

You won't necessarily ask about every item on this list, of course. You may already have some clues from an earlier part of the interview that one of these events is particularly likely. As you ask these questions, remember that correlation does not equal causality. A stressful psychosocial event may have occurred around the time of a psychiatric problem and yet be unrelated to it.

Within the *DSM-IV* system, precipitants would be noted in axis IV, "psychosocial and environmental problems."

LAUNCH INTO THE DIAGNOSTIC QUESTIONS RIGHT AWAY

One of the secrets of efficient and rapid diagnostic interviewing is a gentle tenacity; when the patient mentions a depressed mood, immediately assess for the presence of the diagnostic criteria for depression.

> P: *I think the worst problem over the past couple of weeks is that I've felt so down about myself.*

> I: *Has that down feeling been affecting your sleep?*

> P: *I haven't slept more than 2 or 3 hours a night, and the next day I can barely drag myself to work. I should probably quit anyway; it's a boring job.*

> I: *Have you had problems focusing on your work because of your depression?*

Here, the interviewer stays on the depression topic by cueing off what the patient has said about work (see the discussion of the smooth transition in Chapter 5). If the interviewer had not actively structured the interview this way, the patient might have discussed details of his work environment that would be less relevant to the diagnosis of major depression. Later, when ascertaining the social history, the interviewer can refer to what the patient said about work:

> I: *Earlier, you mentioned that your work is boring. How did you get into that line of work? (Note the use of the referred transition.)*

CURRENT AND PREMORBID LEVEL OF FUNCTIONING

Axis V of the *DSM-IV* diagnostic scheme requests that you note the patient's "GAF," or global assessment of functioning, on a scale of 0 to 100. (See Chapter 31 for more information.) Although I have not found it useful to assign a specific number to functioning, I do think that axis V is an important reminder to the interviewer to ask about both current and baseline functioning. You want to know to what degree your patient's psychiatric illness is impairing her functioning.

To assess overall functioning, ask about the three basic aspects of life: love, work, and fun. *Love* includes all important relationships: family, spouse, and close friends. In addition to paid employment, *work* includes school, volunteer activities, and the structured day activities in which many chronically mentally ill patients participate. *Fun* refers to hobbies and recreational pursuits.

> *How has your illness been affecting your work, relationships, and leisure pursuits?*

The phrasing of this question automatically targets their premorbid functioning. Some patients have a hard time distinguishing a psychiatric illness from the rest of their lives. If so, you will have to follow up with another question to assess their baseline functioning.

> *Before you started to have these anxiety spells (or other symptoms), how was work going?*
>
> *How were you getting along with your family and your wife?*
>
> *What kinds of things were you doing for fun?*

For patients who have more chronic illnesses with multiple exacerbations and remissions, ask the same types of questions about periods between exacerbations:

> *Think about the last time that you were feeling your best, when you weren't hearing any voices and you didn't feel suicidal. How was your life going then? (Follow up with questions about love, work, and fun.)*

Asking about current versus baseline functioning is important diagnostically. The classic example is the difference between schizophrenia and bipolar disorder. In schizophrenia, the patient's level of functioning gradually decreases over months or years, whereas in bipolar disorder, the patient may have been functioning dramatically better within the past few weeks. Determining baseline functioning is also important in setting treatment goals. You might aim to help the patient achieve his best level of functioning over the past year, for example.

CLINICAL VIGNETTE

A resident was working in a busy psychiatric crisis clinic and interviewed a patient who was brought by ambulance for psychotic and disorganized behavior. The patient was a 32-year-old woman and carried the diagnosis of "schizoaffective disorder" in her previous emergency department records. The phrase "history of multiple psychiatric hospitalizations" in the old chart caused the resident to assume that the patient was a chronically poorly functioning woman who could rarely stay out of a hospital. In assessing her psychosocial functioning, the resident was surprised to learn that the patient had been working as a secretary for a research department of a local hospital until 1 year ago, when she had the first of a series of recent hospitalizations. This information caused the resident to pay closer attention to the patient's history and to entertain the possibility of a different diagnosis, such as borderline personality disorder or posttraumatic stress disorder (PTSD), both of which would be more consistent with her good premorbid functioning.

Obtaining the Psychiatric History

13

Essential Questions

Syndromal history:

- How old were you when you first had these symptoms?
- How many episodes have you had?
- When was the last episode?

Mnemonic for treatment history: **G**o **CHaMP**

- **G**eneral questions.
- Who is your current **C**aregiver?
- Have you been psychiatrically **H**ospitalized?
- Have you taken **M**edications for these symptoms?
- Have you had **P**sychotherapy?

Recommended time: 10 minutes

The past psychiatric history (PPH) risks becoming a tedious exercise in documentation. You can avoid this by realizing how vital the PPH is to your twin goals of establishing a diagnosis and formulating a treatment plan.

Specific psychiatric disorders have specific natural histories, with characteristic risk factors, prodromal signs, ages at onset, and prognoses. Obtaining a detailed PPH for a particular patient allows you to compare the course of *her* illness with the textbook's version of the course of illness, increasing the likelihood that you will make a correct diagnosis.

Often patients will come to you after having been treated for many years. One reason such patients are eventually referred to an expert consultant is that experts are great at eliciting a *detailed history of prior treatments*. They can determine exactly what has been tried in the past and whether past treatment trials have been adequate. From this information, they can present informed recommendations about what should be tried next. *And* they can do all this in one or two 50-minute sessions.

Potential pitfalls in obtaining the PPH are similar to those lurking during the HPI. At one end of the continuum, some interviewers get so caught up in the intricacies of the PPH that they spend most of the evaluation time on it, to the detriment of, for example, the PROS. At the other end, the PPH can become a rote exercise and may be obtained too superficially, depriving the interviewer of information necessary to make a firm diagnosis.

OBTAIN THE SYNDROMAL HISTORY

Generally speaking, the HPI will take between 5 and 10 minutes, at the end of which you should have a few provisional diagnoses in mind. Your next job is to obtain the history of these syndromes. Specifically, you want to learn age at onset, premorbid functioning, and history of subsequent episodes up to the present.

• Age at onset:

  How old were you when you first had your symptoms?

  Knowing the age at onset may help you to decide between potential diagnoses, although the most recent epidemiologic data indicate that ages of onset for disorders are less distinct than previously thought (see table below).

Median age at onset of major psychiatric disorders

Disorder	Age (years)
Schizophrenia	21 (men), 27 (women)
Major depression	25
Bipolar disorder	19
Panic disorder	24
Obsessive-compulsive disorder	23
Drug abuse/dependence	18
Alcohol abuse/dependence	21

Adapted from Burke, J. D., and Reiger, D. A. (1994). Epidemiology of mental disorders. In R. E. Hales, S. C. Yudofsky, and J. A. Talbott (Eds.), *American Psychiatric Press Textbook of Psychiatry*. Washington, DC: American Psychiatric Press, 19.

• Premorbid functioning/baseline functioning: See Chapter 12 for a discussion of this.

- History and precipitants of subsequent episodes up to present: Include questions about the severity of episodes and exacerbations, as well as the duration of episodes. Often, this information comes out when you are obtaining the treatment history. For example, episodes of mania or exacerbations of schizophrenia often correspond with hospitalizations.

  As with hospitalizations, a time-efficient method of asking about episodes is to ask about the first one, the latest one, and the total number of episodes.

  When did you have your first breakdown?

  How many have you had total?

  When was your last one?

OBTAIN THE TREATMENT HISTORY

You ask about prior treatments mostly to help with future treatment decisions but also to help nail down a diagnosis. For example, if lithium was helpful for an affective episode, bipolar disorder would be high on your list. You want to know what has been tried in the past and whether it has worked. Accuracy and detail are important here, because a sloppy treatment history can lead to poor future treatment decisions. For example, patients may be falsely labeled "treatment resistant" on the basis of old records indicating that numerous medications were "tried but were unsuccessful." On closer questioning, such patients may in fact have had few adequate trials of medication.

I suggest the following format for obtaining the treatment history:

General questions

Current caregivers

Hospitalization history

Medication history

Psychotherapy history

Use the mnemonic Go CHaMP so that you don't miss any category.

You won't necessarily ask your questions in the above order—in fact, you will obtain much of this information during the HPI—but it's helpful to think about these five aspects of the treatment history to make sure that you haven't neglected to ask important questions. At some point during the interview, mentally review whether you have obtained enough information about each of these categories.

General Questions

What sort of treatment have you had for your depression?

What was the most helpful?

More sophisticated and forthcoming patients will tell you almost everything you need to know about the treatment history in response to a general question. Other patients will require more specific questioning.

What was going on in your life during the period when you were depression-free?

In some cases, the best "treatment" for a particular patient was a close relationship with someone or their escape from a dysfunctional relationship. You can learn this from a careful history, and it may become a part of your treatment recommendations.

Current Caregivers

You will need to know who your patient is seeing currently. If he is a new patient, you may be the only caregiver. If you are interviewing a patient with a chronic mental illness, he will likely have both a therapist and a psychopharmacologist, and he may also have a case worker (usually a social worker), a group therapist, and a primary care doctor (a family practitioner or an internist) and may be involved in day treatment or residential treatment.

Hospitalization History

Have you ever been hospitalized for a psychiatric problem?

For patients who have had multiple hospitalizations, do not spend your time ascertaining the names of the hospitals and dates of each admission; this could take the entire 50 minutes. Instead, find out when they were first and last hospitalized and about how many hospitalizations they've had over their lifetime. If a patient has had many hospitalizations, try to find out if they are clustered around a specific few years. Some patients will have had several hospitalizations earlier in the course of their disorder because they had little insight into their problem and were noncompliant with their medications. Later in life, their hospitalizations may be spaced much further apart. Alternatively, the opposite pattern may appear, in which an affective disorder worsens with age. Think of hospitalizations as markers of disease severity.

> *When were you first hospitalized?*
>
> *How many hospitalizations have you had in your life?*
>
> *How many have you had in the past year?*
>
> *When was your last hospitalization?*

In addition to asking these questions, it is often useful to ask why your patient was hospitalized:

> *In general, what sorts of things have caused you to need to be in the hospital?*

Your assumptions about reason for hospitalization may be wrong, as illustrated by the following example.

CLINICAL VIGNETTE

A patient with chronic schizophrenia stated that he'd been hospitalized several times over the past 2 years. The resident initially assumed that these hospitalizations were for psychotic decompensations, but when asked, the patient said that most were alcohol detox admissions. This prompted the resident to obtain a much more thorough substance abuse history than he had planned.

Ask how the patient has benefited (or suffered) from hospitalizations:

> *Have your hospitalizations been helpful for you? Why (or why not)?*

The answer to this question is often highly informative. It may clue you in to the degree of insight that the patient has into the illness. ("They treated me like a prisoner. There was no reason for me to be there," implies relatively little insight, for example.) It may also give you a sense of when the patient needs to be hospitalized. For some patients, a relatively early, brief hospitalization at the first signs of decompensation can avert a much worse episode.

Medication History

The most important limit on the bioavailability of medication has nothing to do with pharmacodynamics or pharmacokinetics; rather, it is patient non-compliance.

Dr. Ross Baldessarini
Chief of Psychopharmacology
McLean Hospital

Have you been on medications for your depression?

To the extent possible, document all the medications the patient has tried. Many patients will not remember generic names or may only remember what the pill looked like or the side effect it caused. Obviously, the more you know about alternative names, shapes, and side effects of medication, the more efficiently you will be able to obtain this history. I find it helpful to have a *Physician's Desk Reference* (PDR) at my side, because it has photographs of many medications, to help patients identify them. For psychologists and social workers, a number of books have been published that teach the basics of psychopharmacology to non-MDs, and I recommend that you become familiar with this information.

For how many weeks did you take your medications?

Many psychiatric medications take several weeks to have a therapeutic effect. Antidepressants take 4 to 6 weeks. Antipsychotics may take 1 to 2 weeks or longer, depending on the clinical situation. Thus, merely documenting that a patient has tried a particular medication does not mean that he's had an *adequate* trial.

At this point, a normalizing question may be helpful:

> *Often, people do not necessarily take their medications every day, but will take them every so often, depending on how they feel. Was that true for you?*

Some patients will say that they took their medication for months or years, but on close questioning, you will find that they only took it once a week or so. This may have been because of side effects or because they were under the mistaken impression that they were only supposed to take their medication when they felt depressed or lethargic.

Or a behavior expectation question may be appropriate:

> *What sorts of side effects did you have on the medication?*

Almost all patients experience at least some side effects with medications, and it's important to document them so that a bothersome side effect can be avoided in the future.

> *What medication was most helpful?*
>
> *What was least helpful?*

CLINICAL VIGNETTE

A resident was doing a psychopharmacologic evaluation of a 46-year-old married Latino woman with a several-year history of depression and anxiety. During the treatment history, the patient stated that she had taken a number of different antidepressants from different classes with only minimal effectiveness. The resident asked a normalizing question about whether the patient had taken her medications consistently; she responded that she only took them when she felt anxious, which varied from daily to once every 2 weeks. In fact, the resident was unable to document an adequate trial of *any* antidepressant and subsequently focused on educating the patient on the necessity of consistently taking medications.

Psychotherapy History

In recent years, psychotherapies have become increasingly tailored to specific disorders, and evidence of effectiveness has become irrefutable (Barlow 1993). In addition, it has become clear that therapy can have negative side effects, as can medication. Thus, obtaining a history of psychotherapeutic treatments is important.

> *Have you ever had counseling or therapy for your problem?*
>
> *How often did you see your therapist?*
>
> *How long did you see him/her?*

These basic parameters of session frequency and length of treatment are usually nonthreatening and easy to elicit.

> *What sort of therapy did you have?*
>
> *Did it have a name, like "cognitive therapy," "behavior therapy," or "psychodynamic therapy"?*

More often than not, your patient will not know the technical name of the therapy he received. You can compensate for this by describing the therapy.

> *Did your therapist focus on "automatic thoughts" that make you more anxious or depressed?*
>
> *Did she give you homework assignments between sessions?*
>
> *Did she have you practice doing things that caused you anxiety? (For cognitive-behavioral therapy.)*
>
> *Did your therapist focus on your childhood experiences and how those affect your current life? (For psychodynamic therapy.)*

You can also ask a more open-ended question:

> *Without going into too much detail, what sorts of things did you focus on in therapy?*
>
> *Was your therapist a psychologist, a psychiatrist, or a social worker?*

Knowing this may or may not be useful. For example, a patient may say she had a therapist, when in fact she was seen by a psychiatrist once a month for brief visits. This was more likely psychopharmacologic management than psychotherapy.

> *How did you like working with your therapist?*
>
> *Was the therapy helpful?*
>
> *In what ways was it helpful?*

This information will be particularly valuable in assessing the patient's suitability for further therapy.

> *How did you leave treatment?*

The way a patient ended treatment may tell you much about how he viewed treatment and may help you plan how to proceed with your own treatment of the patient. Some patients, for instance, have a history of ending therapy by simply not showing up for the next session. Others may have had a stormy termination. Others may have terminated "by the book" but continue to feel unexpressed sad or angry feelings toward the therapist.

14 ▼ Screening for General Medical Conditions

> ### Screening Questions
> Mnemonic: **MIDAS**
> - Do you take any **M**edications now?
> - Do you have any medical **I**llnesses?
> - Do you have a primary care **D**octor?
> - Have you ever had **A**llergies, reactions, or side effects from any medications?
> - Have you ever had any **S**urgery?
>
> Medical Review of Systems
>
> *Recommended time:* 3 minutes

There are two major reasons for asking about the medical history in psychiatric patients:

- **To screen for medical illnesses.** Many psychiatric patients, particularly chronic schizophrenics in public care systems, have very poor medical follow-up, both because they are indigent and because their psychiatric disorder leads to poor compliance with appointments (Hall et al. 1980). Thus, they may have a high prevalence of undiagnosed medical conditions. Whether these conditions affect their psychiatric status or not, you will do them a large service by screening for medical conditions for which they may not be receiving treatment.
- **To uncover general medical causes of psychiatric illness.** A number of medical illnesses and medications can cause psychiatric syndromes and aggravate preexisting ones (Lishman 1987). This is a convenient section of the interview for asking about such illnesses.

MIDAS

If you can develop the **MIDAS** touch, you'll never forget to ask about the medical history:

Medications

Illness history

80

Primary care Doctor

Allergies

Surgical history

Medications

Obtain a list of all medications, including those for general medical conditions. Ascertain whether the patient has been taking them as prescribed (see Chapter 11).

History of Medical Illnesses

You can begin with a screening question such as

Do you have any medical problems?

Have you ever had a medical illness?

However, a common problem with this approach occurs when the patient says "no" without thinking carefully, as the following vignette illustrates.

CLINICAL VIGNETTE

A 36-year-old woman with several past hospitalizations for depression was asked if she had any medical problems, to which she replied, "No." Later, when the resident asked what medications she took, she listed a number of psychotropics and then said, "and I also take Synthroid." The resident said, "I thought you had no medical problems," to which the patient replied, "I don't. I used to have hypothyroidism, but that was corrected with the Synthroid."

Primary Care Doctor

In the preceding vignette, asking about illness elicited invalid information. One way to increase the validity of your medical history questions is to first ask if the patient is being seen by a doctor.

Do you see a doctor regularly?

What does he/she treat you for?

By referring to a relationship with a caregiver, you will typically jog the patient's memory for past diagnoses and treatments. You can also learn information about the patient's character:

I: *Do you see a doctor regularly?*

P: *Yeah, I see someone at the clinic. Not that he gives a damn about me.*

Such a statement could be explored further and might be a clue to character traits that may interfere with treatment, such as passive-aggressive or self-defeating traits.

While you're at it, ask the patient if you may contact his doctor to share information. Discussing the patient with the primary care physician will help round out your evaluation, as well as provide useful information to the caregiver who referred the patient to you.

Allergies

The usual screening question is

Do you have allergies to any medications?

This may work, but again there are potential pitfalls. Some patients have idiosyncratic understandings of what constitutes an allergy. They may think you're asking about serious allergic reactions, such as bronchospasm, and therefore may answer in the negative even if they've had milder allergic reactions. They also may not realize that you're interested in hearing about any negative reactions to medications, and not just allergies per se. Better to ask

Have you ever had any allergies, reactions, or side effects to any medication?

A patient may say that he is allergic to a number of medications that only uncommonly produce true allergic reactions, such as neuroleptics and antidepressants. If so, pursue the nature of the allergy.

What kinds of reactions did you have to that medicine?

If the patient's response is vague, make some suggestions based on your knowledge of drug effects:

Did the Haldol give you muscle spasms? Did it make your hands shake or your body move slowly?

When you document allergies in your write-up, specify the nature of the reaction. For example, writing that a patient is "allergic to neuroleptics" is probably inaccurate and might mean that the patient will never again be offered a neuroleptic, even if she could benefit from it. A more accurate statement would be, "Haldol causes dystonia." This leaves the door open to trials of other neuroleptics.

Surgical History

It is important to ask specifically about previous surgery; many patients do not volunteer this information when asked about "medical problems," either because it was too long ago or because they do not consider an operation to have indicated a medical problem per se.

CLINICAL VIGNETTE

A 54-year-old man with major depression had mentioned gastritis as his only medical problem. Midway through the interview, he mentioned in passing, "I divorced my wife back in '84 or so, just after they took out part of my pancreas." On further exploration, the patient considered that operation to be a turning point in his life, because he made the decision to stop drinking then and had been sober since.

MEDICAL REVIEW OF SYSTEMS

The purpose of the review of symptoms is to note medical problems that the patient may have forgotten to describe in response to the MIDAS questions. Whether it's necessary to do a review of symptoms for every patient is a matter of controversy. The MIDAS questions may miss seemingly minor symptoms that may be the first clues to a big problem, such as the occasional cough that signals lung cancer. But the review of symptoms takes a lot of time, and most mental health clinicians refer their patients to an internist for physical examinations anyway.

Here's a compromise. I'll outline two approaches to the review of symptoms, a brief review of symptoms (1 minute) and a more extended one (5 minutes). Which approach is better depends on the patient and the clinical setting.

Brief versus full review of symptoms

Review of symptoms	Patient	Rationale
Brief	Young, middle or upper class	Statistically, fewer medical problems; good follow-up with doctors
Full	Elderly	Statistically, more medical problems
	Chronically mentally ill	Poor follow-up with doctors

Both the brief and extended reviews of symptoms begin with systemic questions and progress in head-to-toe order, which is an easy way to remember them and to ensure that you do not forget to ask important questions.

Brief Review of Systems

I'm going to ask whether you're having problems with various parts of your body, moving from your head to your toes. Any problems with headaches or seizures? Vision or hearing problems? Smelling, taste, or throat problems? Thyroid problems? Problems with your lungs like pneumonia or coughing? Heart problems? Stomach problems like ulcers or constipation? Problems with urination? Joint problems? Problems walking?

Extended Review of Systems
General

Overall, do you feel healthy?

Do you have joint problems or skin problems? (May indicate systemic lupus.)

Do you have excessive bleeding or anemia? (Anemia can cause depression.)

Do you have diabetes or thyroid problems? (Diabetes can cause lethargy; thyroid problems can cause depression or mania.)

Have you ever had cancer?

Do you have any infections, such as HIV or tuberculosis (TB)? (HIV can mimic many psychiatric disorders; TB can mimic depression.)

HEENT (Head, Eyes, Ears, Nose, and Throat)

Do you get headaches? (Can be caused by brain tumor.)

Have you ever had a head injury? (Can lead to neuropsychiatric conditions.)

Any problems with your vision or your hearing?

Do you ever see or hear things that other people don't notice? (Provides a convenient place to ask about psychotic phenomena in a nonthreatening way.)

Do you get nosebleeds?

Do you smell things that other people don't? (Often a sign of temporal lobe epilepsy.)

How are your teeth?

Do you often get sore throats?

Cardiovascular and Respiratory

Do you have any heart problems?

Do you have chest pains; do you have palpitations of your heart?

Do you have high blood pressure?

Do you experience shortness of breath (emphysema, coronary artery disease)?

Do you cough excessively (lung cancer)?

Do you wheeze (asthma)?

NOTES

Differentiate panic attack from cardiac disease; rule out congestive heart failure as a cause of lethargy and fatigue that might be mistakenly diagnosed as depression. Look for diagnostic clues to the presence of lung cancer, which can mimic the anorexia and weight loss of depression.

Gastrointestinal

> *Do you have problems with nausea or vomiting?*
>
> *Do you ever make yourself vomit? (A screen for bulimic behavior.)*
>
> *Do you have problems swallowing?*
>
> *Do you have constipation or diarrhea?*
>
> *Have you noticed any change in your stool?*

NOTES

Rule out hidden colon or stomach cancer; diagnose irritable bowel syndrome, which often accompanies psychiatric complaints. Answers to these questions may provide direction in the choice of medications (e.g., you'd want to avoid a tricyclic antidepressant in a patient with preexisting constipation).

Genitourinary and Gynecologic

> *Do you have problems with urination, such as burning or excessive urination?*
>
> *Do you have retention of urine or incontinence?*
>
> *Do you have any problems with sexual functioning or sexual drive?*
>
> *Have you ever had a venereal disease (HIV, syphilis)?*
>
> *When were your last pap smear and mammogram?*
>
> *Do you have any problems with menstruation? When was your last menstrual period?*
>
> *Might you be pregnant?*

NOTES

Rule out bladder cancer; prostate cancer in men; and uterine, ovarian, or breast cancer in women. Establish amenorrhea of anorexia nervosa. Determine contraindications to the use of anticholinergic medications, such as an enlarged prostate.

Neurologic

Have you had seizures?

Have you ever passed out?

Have you ever had a stroke?

Any tingling in your arms or legs?

Any problems with walking, coordination, and balance?

Any problems talking or thinking?

Any changes in your handwriting?

NOTES

Detect brain tumor, epilepsy, stroke. Screen for multiple sclerosis, Parkinson's disease, and dementia.

Assessing HIV Risk. *

I've set up a separate category for HIV risk because it's particularly important, and it can be an awkward subject to bring up. Later in the interview, during the social history, you'll ask some questions about intimate relationships to assess your patient's capacity for relatedness. Here, you focus on sexual functioning as it relates to risk of HIV, but this may lead to a discussion of other concerns.

Begin with an introductory statement such as

> *Here are some questions I routinely ask. Some may be uncomfortable; let me know if they are.*

> *If I may, I'd like to ask you some sexual history questions, because many people are concerned about AIDS.*

Then, go on to the screening questions for HIV:

> *Are you sexually active, or have you ever injected drugs, even once?*

> *Do you have any reason to believe you are at risk for HIV?*

Follow the preceding questions, depending on whether you are talking to a man or woman, with these:

---

*I thank Stephen Brady, Ph.D., for suggesting many of these questions.

> *(For men): Have you had sex with a man in the past 15 years? (If yes): Can I ask what kind of sex that was? Was it oral sex or anal sex? Did you use a condom?*

> *(For women): Have you had sex with a man who sleeps with other men or who injects drugs?*

> *(For both men and women): How many sexual partners have you had over the past year?*

At this point, you've done an adequate assessment for HIV risk. You may want to follow up with some general questions about sexual functioning, which is often affected by psychiatric disorders and by the medications used to treat them.

> *Are you satisfied with your sexual functioning?*

> *Do you find that your sexual functioning changes when you get depressed (or substitute other relevant psychiatric symptom)?*

If you are interviewing someone who you suspect has been sexually abused or raped, this is a good time to ask about it.

> *Sometimes people have sex against their will. Has that ever happened to you?*

> *Have you ever been coerced into having sex?*

 NOTES

These questions avoid the loaded terms *rape*, *molest*, and *abuse*. This is useful for patients who have been sexually coerced by a spouse or a relative and who may not want to think of their experiences in such terms.

Family Psychiatric History

Screening Questions

- Has any blood relative ever had nervousness, a nervous breakdown, depression, mania, psychosis or schizophrenia, alcohol or drug abuse, suicide attempts, or hospitalization for nervousness?
- Has any blood relative ever had a medical or neurologic illness such as heart disease, diabetes, cancer, seizures, or senility?

Recommended time: 2 minutes for bare bones; 5 minutes for genogram

The family history may be approached in one of two ways. One is the bare-bones approach, which aims to ascertain the patient's inherited risk of developing a psychiatric or medical disorder. The second approach is more extensive and is a way of beginning the social history part of the interview. I describe both approaches here and let you decide which works best for you.

BARE-BONES APPROACH

Ask the following long, high-yield question, which is adapted from a question suggested by Morrison and Munoz (1991, p. 102):

> *Has any blood relative ever had nervousness, nervous breakdown, depression, mania, psychosis or schizophrenia, alcohol or drug abuse, suicide attempts, or hospitalization for nervousness?*

Because the question is so long, you have to ask it very slowly, pausing after each disorder so that the patient has time to think about it. You should also define *blood relative.*

> *By blood relative, I mean parents, brothers, sisters, uncles, aunts, grandparents, and cousins.*

HOT TIP

If the patient answers with a definitive "no," you can move on. If there was a "yes," you should try to determine exactly what the diagnosis was. Unless your patient is in the mental health field and is familiar with its jargon, this may not be easy. It's helpful to ask about specific treatments the relative may have received, such as lithium, carbamazepine (Tegretol), divalproex sodium (Depakote) (clues to bipolar disorder), neuroleptics [ask about haloperidol (Haldol) and chlorpromazine (Thorazine), since they were widely used in the past], electroconvulsive therapy (clue to depression, bipolar disorder, or schizophrenia, depending on when the treatment was administered), antidepressants, and antianxiety agents. Remember that medications were used differently 20 years ago. For example, in its heyday, diazepam (Valium) was given to many patients for depression, whereas now a history of benzodiazepine treatment is a clue for the presence of an anxiety disorder.

To determine a family history of transmissible medical and neurologic problems, ask

> *Has any blood relative ever had a medical or neurologic illness, such as heart disease, diabetes, cancer, seizures, or senility?*

How does it help diagnostically to know that a patient has a first-degree relative with a psychiatric disorder? The table below lists those psychiatric disorders for which there is significant evidence of familial transmission. The relative risk compares the risk for people with such a family history against the risk of people in the general population, who are assigned a relative risk of 1.0. For example, the relative risk of developing bipolar disorder is 25; this means that if your patient's father is bipolar, she is 25 times more likely to develop bipolar disorder than the average person. The baseline lifetime prevalence of each disorder is also listed in the table.

Typically, family information is used in conjunction with other clinical information. For example, family history is crucial in deciding whether a patient with new-onset psychosis has schizophrenia or is in the manic phase of bipolar disorder.

Psychiatric disorders with significant evidence of familial transmission

DSM-IV disorder	Lifetime relative risk if first-degree relative has disorder[a]	Lifetime prevalence in general population[b]
Bipolar disorder	25	1
Schizophrenia	19	1
Bulimia nervosa	10	2[c]
Panic disorder	10	4
Alcoholism	7	14
Generalized anxiety disorder	6	5
Anorexia nervosa	5	1[c]
Specific phobia	3	11
Social phobia	3	13
Somatization disorder	3	2[d]
Major depression	3	17
Obsessive-compulsive disorder	?	3[e]
Agoraphobia	3	5

[a]Relative risk figures from Reider, R. O., Kaufmann, C. A., et al. (1994). Genetics. In R. E. Hales, S. C. Yudofsky and J. A. Talbott (Eds.), *American Psychiatric Press Textbook of Psychiatry*. Washington, DC: American Psychiatric Press. See text for explanation.

[b]Lifetime prevalence figures from Kessler, R. C., McGonagle, K. A., Zhao, S., Nelson, C. B., Hughes, M., Eshleman, S., Wittchen, H. U., and Kendler, K. S. (1994). Lifetime and 12-month prevalence of DSM-III-R psychiatric disorders in the United States. *Archives of General Psychiatry, 51,* 8–19; and Regier, D. A., Farmer, M. E., et al. (1990). Comorbidity of mental disorders with alcohol and other drug abuse. *Journal of the American Medical Association, 264,* 2511–2518.

[c]From Halmi, K. A. (1994). Eating disorders: Anorexia nervosa, bulimia nervosa, and obesity. In R. E. Hales, S. C. Yudofsky, and J. A. Talbott (Eds.), *American Psychiatric Press Textbook of Psychiatry*. Washington, DC: American Psychiatric Press.

[d]From Martin, R. L., and Yutzy, S. H. (1994). Somatoform disorders. In R. E. Hales, S. C. Yudofsky, and J. A. Talbott (Eds.), *American Psychiatric Press Textbook of Psychiatry*. Washington, DC: American Psychiatric Press.

[e]From Hollander, E., Simeon, D., et al. (1994). Anxiety disorders. In R. E. Hales, S. C. Yudofsky, and J. A. Talbott (Eds.), *American Psychiatric Press Textbook of Psychiatry*. Washington, DC: American Psychiatric Press.

THE GENOGRAM:
FAMILY HISTORY AS SOCIAL HISTORY

Doing a genogram takes a while, which probably explains its lack of popularity in most clinical settings. But it doesn't take *that* long, and the time investment usually pays off in terms of richness of information. The genogram serves the additional function of introducing you to the patient's developmental history.

The technique is simple. Begin by telling your patient that you'd like to draw a family diagram in order to better understand her family. Draw small squares for males and circles for females. Obtain the following information about each relative:

- Age
- If dead, year, age, and cause of death (put slash mark through square or circle if dead)
- Presence of psychiatric problem, substance abuse, or major medical problem
- Status of the patient's relationship with relative (e.g., close, estranged, a perpetrator or victim of sexual or physical abuse)

Begin by diagramming the first-degree relatives, with the oldest sibling on the right.

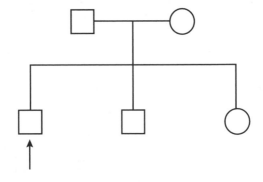

Once you have the skeleton of the chart, ask about each family member and embellish the chart with the information obtained. While you will likely develop your own preferences, it is standard to write the age within the circle or square, to use slashes to represent the deceased, and to use double slashes to represent a divorce. In this example, the patient is a divorced 34-year-old man with two children who has a family psychiatric history significant for alcoholism and depression.

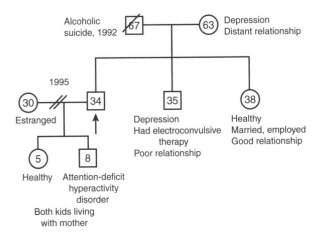

Once you have completed a genogram, you have accomplished three tasks: You have obtained (a) the family psychiatric history, (b) the family medical history, and (c) the bare bones of the social and developmental history. Also, the physical layout of the genogram makes it a quick way to remind yourself of the patient's social situation, a particularly nice feature if you rarely see the patient.

16 Obtaining the Social and Developmental History

Essential Questions

- Can you tell me a bit about your background, where you grew up, and how you grew up?
- Explore the following topics chronologically:
  Early family life
  School experiences, emphasizing friendships
  Work experiences
  Intimate relationships and sexual history
  Current social support network
  Goals and aspirations

Recommended time: 5 minutes

What's the purpose of the social and developmental history in a brief diagnostic interview? How extensive should it be? The social history is useful in two closely related ways: (a) It allows you to get to know the patient as a *person* rather than as a *diagnosis*, and (b) you can approach the diagnosis of a personality disorder through the social history (see Chapter 28).

The essential questions take 5 minutes to ask, whereas the extended version takes 10 to 20 minutes and should be reserved for occasions on which you can take two sessions to do the evaluation.

EARLY FAMILY LIFE

Begin with the following introductory question:

> *Can you tell me a bit about your background, where you grew up, and how you grew up?*

Proceed to more specific questions, moving chronologically through the stages of life.

> *How many siblings did you have, and where were you in the birth order?*

Each family configuration has a unique impact on psychological development. Typical scenarios include the loneliness of the only child, the eldest child of a large family who was forced into the role of a parent, the ignored middle child, and the youngest child who grew up as the resented apple of his mother's eye.

> *What did your parents do for a living?*

Parental employment may have affected the patient's relationship with her parents. For example, a father who worked as a traveling salesman may not have been home much. This question also gives you a sense of socioeconomic situation: Did the patient grow up amid poverty or affluence?

> *How did you get along with your parents?*

Although there's not enough time to do this topic justice in the diagnostic interview, these questions will give you an idea of the general flavor of the home. Was it a peaceful, loving environment, or was it angry and chaotic?

> *What did they do when you disobeyed?*

This question can gently introduce the topic of physical or sexual abuse. Depending on the answer, you can follow up with a more explicit question, such as

> *Were you abused physically or sexually as you grew up?*

> *Were there any other important adults in the home?*

Often, another relative was a major factor in the patient's early life, with either a positive or a negative effect.

> *How did you get along with your siblings?*

A close relationship with siblings can often compensate for a terrible relationship with parents.

> *Who were you closest to, growing up?*

EDUCATION AND WORK

> *Did you enjoy school?*

This question will give you a sense of how the patient managed her first encounter with the social field outside of the family.

> *Did you have many friends, or did you keep to yourself?*

> *Did you have a best friend?*

The patient's lifelong pattern of relating is often apparent in the first few years of school.

> *What kinds of grades did you get?*

Grades are a rough measure of intelligence and perseverance.

> *What did you do after you graduated (or dropped out)?*

Did she take the straight and narrow course to college or into the job world? Or did she wander for a while, not certain what to do with her life?

> *Did you like your work?*
>
> *How well did you get along with employers and colleagues?*

Did the patient's pattern of relating continue unaltered as she entered the work environment? Did she have any difficulties dealing with authority figures?

INTIMATE RELATIONSHIPS (SEXUAL HISTORY)

How does one ask about sexuality? It's always an awkward topic, and patients are usually guarded about revealing sexual information, especially when it pertains to sexual orientation. One study showed that adolescents are four times more likely to reveal a history of homosexual contact to a computer than to a person, but even the responses revealed to the computer were well below estimates of the actual prevalence of homosexuality in adolescents (Turner et al. 1996). Thus, asking about sexual history requires extra sensitivity.

Recall that in Chapter 12, I suggested some sexual history questions in the context of the medical history and the assessment of the risk for HIV. An alternative tactic is to approach these issues from within the social history. Here, the rationale for obtaining a sexual history is not so much to assess HIV risk as it is to assess the quality of the patient's intimate relationships. Is she capable of relating intimately with another? Are her intimate relationships stable or transient and chaotic, as in the case of patients with borderline personality disorder?

As with the rest of the social history, proceed chronologically:

> *When did you first begin dating?*

Eventually, you'll decide on a way of asking about sexual orientation that is comfortable for you. The trick is to be nonjudgmental.

Were you attracted to men, women, or both?

The above question should be asked in a very matter-of-fact way, with the unspoken message that it will not faze you if the patient says that he is attracted to the same sex.

Other options are as follows:

- Precede your question with a normalizing statement, such as: "Adolescents often experiment with different sexual lifestyles; was that true for you? What's your current sexual preference?"
- At the beginning of the interview, slip your question into a checklist of routine questions: "How old are you? What's your marital status? And your sexual preference?"
- Ask during the medical history when you ask about risk factors for HIV: "Do you have any risk factors for the HIV virus? Have you had homosexual sex?"

> *Are you satisfied with your sex life?*
>
> *Are there things about your sex life or your sexual desires that make you uncomfortable?*
>
> *When did you have your first important relationship?*
>
> *What attracted you to that person?*

Is the patient capable of establishing an intimate relationship? Can he describe other people in three-dimensional terms?

CLINICAL VIGNETTE

An attending clinician was interviewing a 40-year-old divorced man in the hospital for depression. His wife and daughter had left him 2 years earlier. He had a lifelong pattern of brief and shallow relationships. The following exchange took place as the attending clinician was exploring the relationship history:

> I: *Tell me about your girlfriends.*
>
> P: *They were animals.*
>
> I: *Pick one, and tell me about her.*
>
> P: *I met a woman last year; she was a stray cat.*
>
> I: *Why do you say she was a stray cat?*
>
> P: *She had no connections.*

I: *What was it that you were attracted to?*

P: *Her body.*

I: *Okay. What kicked in about her personality later?*

P: *What do you mean?*

I: *If I met her, what would I notice about her?*

P: *It's tough to answer. Her attitude.*

I: *How was that?*

P: *It was good.*

The patient was unable to discuss any important person in his life in more than a superficial way, which mirrored his fears of intimacy.

CURRENT ACTIVITIES AND RELATIONSHIPS

What attracted you to your current significant other?

How has your marriage (relationship) gone?

Do you have any close friends (aside from your spouse)?

Are you in touch with your family?

Does the patient have a social support system in place? Who would she call if she were in trouble?

What do you do during your leisure time?

Does she enjoy sports, hobbies, reading, going to movies, and other activities, or does she only work?

What do you think you'll be doing 5 years from now, and what would you like to be doing?

This question provides a window into the patient's view of her future and her dreams and aspirations.

CLINICAL VIGNETTE

An attending clinician was interviewing a 32-year-old single woman who had worked as an extremely successful attorney until a year ago, when she was fired while in the middle of a major depression. During the social history, she related that she disliked physicians in general, because her abusive father was a physician.

Toward the end of the interview, the attending clinician asked

> I: *What do you think you'll be doing in 5 years, and what would you like to be doing?*
>
> P: *I'll probably be dead. I'd like to be a physician.*

The attending clinician then productively explored the meaning of her seemingly paradoxical desire to become a physician.

INTERVIEWING FOR DIAGNOSIS: THE PSYCHIATRIC REVIEW OF SYMPTOMS

It takes two to tell the truth:
One to say it and one to hear it.

Henry David Thoreau

How to Memorize the *DSM-IV*

> **Essential Concepts**
>
> **DSM-IV Mnemonic:**
> **D**epressed **P**atients **S**ound **A**nxious,
> **S**o **C**laim **P**sychiatrists.
> - **D**epression and other mood disorders
> - **P**sychotic disorders
> - **S**ubstance abuse disorders
> - **A**nxiety disorders
> - **S**omatoform disorders
> - **C**ognitive disorders
> - **P**ersonality disorders

Everything should be as simple as it is, but not simpler.

Albert Einstein

In this chapter, I describe an approach to memorizing the criteria for the major *DSM-IV* disorders. These mnemonics are a way of sorting information into manageable chunks. Those who have researched the way expert clinicians think have found that this "chunking" process is quite common (Kaplan 1995). The father of chunking, Miller (1957), showed that humans can only process about 7 (±2) bits of information at a time, which is, presumably, why phone numbers have seven digits. You have to be able to process more than seven items to master the *DSM-IV*, but mnemonics help, by grouping items into information-packed chunks.

MEMORIZE THE SEVEN
MAJOR DIAGNOSTIC CATEGORIES

Begin by mastering the following mnemonic for the seven major adult diagnostic categories in the *DSM-IV*:

Depressed Patients Sound Anxious, So Claim Psychiatrists

Depression and other mood disorders (major depression, bipolar disorder, dysthymia)

Psychotic disorders (schizophrenia, schizoaffective disorder, delusional disorder)

Substance abuse disorders (alcohol and drug abuse, psychiatric syndromes induced by drug and alcohol use)

Anxiety disorders [panic disorder, agoraphobia, generalized anxiety disorder (GAD), obsessive-compulsive disorder (OCD)]

Somatoform disorders (somatization disorder, eating disorders)

Cognitive disorders (dementia, mental retardation, ADHD)

Personality disorders

Notice that these categories deviate somewhat from *DSM-IV* dogma. For example, I call ADHD a "cognitive disorder," whereas the *DSM-IV* classifies it as a "disorder of infancy, childhood, and adolescence." Also, I classify eating disorders under somatoform disorders, whereas the *DSM-IV* puts them in a separate chapter. My purpose here is not to create a new classification of psychiatric disorders but simply to rearrange them into seven categories for ease of memorization.

FOCUS ON POSITIVE CRITERIA

Now that you've memorized the major disorders, you need to memorize the diagnostic criteria. Begin by disregarding the voluminous exclusions and modifiers listed by the *DSM-IV* and instead focus on the actual behaviors and affects needed to make the diagnosis.

For example, under schizophrenia in the *DSM-IV* are six categories of criteria, labeled *A* through *F*. *B* is the usual proviso that the disorder must cause significant dysfunction, which is true for all the disorders, so you don't need to memorize it. *D* tells you to rule out schizoaffective and mood disorder before you diagnose schizophrenia—another obvious piece of information; don't use up valuable neurons memorizing it. *E* reminds you to rule out substance abuse or a medical condition, which you should do before making any diagnosis, and *F* deals with the arcane issue of diagnosing schizophrenia in someone who's autistic. So, only two essential criteria are left: *A* (symptoms) and *C* (duration).

This section lists mnemonics for most of the major disorders, but it does not cover how to ascertain the diagnoses, which involves the skillful use of probing questions and specific follow-up questions. These are covered in detail in Chapters 21–28, where the full *DSM-IV* criteria are spelled out.

✡ KEY POINT

How should you use these mnemonics? They are primarily an aid to ensure that you remember to ask about major diagnostic criteria. Do not ask the questions in the same order as the mnemonics; doing so would lead to a very stilted interview. Try to ask diagnostic questions when they seem to fit naturally into the context of the interview, using some of the techniques for making transitions already discussed in Chapters 4 and 6.

Unless stated otherwise, these mnemonics are the products of my own disordered brain.

Mood Disorders

Major Depression: SIGECAPS.   Four out of these eight, with depressed mood or anhedonia, for 2 weeks signify major depression:

Sleep disorder (either increased or decreased sleep)

Interest deficit (anhedonia)

Guilt (worthlessness, hopelessness, regret)

Energy deficit

Concentration deficit

Appetite disorder (either decreased or increased appetite)

Psychomotor retardation or agitation

Suicidality

This mnemonic, devised by Dr. Cary Gross of the Massachusetts General Hospital Department of Psychiatry, refers to what might be written on a prescription sheet for a depressed, anergic patient: SIG: Energy CAPSules. Each letter refers to one of the major diagnostic criteria for a major depressive disorder. To meet the criteria for an episode of major depression, your patient must have had four of the preceding symptoms and depressed mood or anhedonia for at least 2 weeks.

Dysthymia: ACHEWS.   Two out of these six, with depressed mood, for 2 years signify dysthymia:

Appetite disorder (either decreased or increased)

Concentration deficit

Hopelessness

Energy deficit

Worthlessness

Sleep disorder (either increased or decreased)

The dysthymic patient is "allergic" to happiness; hence, the mnemonic refers to a dysthymic patient's (misspelled) sneezes (achoos) on exposure to happiness. To meet the criteria, the patient must have had 2 years of depressed mood with two of the six symptoms in the mnemonic.

Manic Episode: DIGFAST.   Elevated mood with three of these seven, or irritable mood with four of these seven, for 1 week signify a manic episode:

Distractibility

Indiscretion (*DSM-IV*'s "excessive involvement in pleasurable activities . . .")

Grandiosity

Flight of ideas

Activity increase

Sleep deficit (decreased need for sleep)

Talkativeness (pressured speech)

I don't know who came up with this jewel, but I use it all the time. *DIGFAST* apparently refers to the speed with which a manic patient would dig a hole if put to the task. A complication in the diagnosis is that if the mood is primarily irritable, four of seven criteria must be met to qualify.

Psychotic Disorders

Schizophrenia: Delusions Herald Schizophrenic's Bad News.   Two of these five for 1 month, with 5 months prodromal or residual symptoms, signify schizophrenia:

Delusions

Hallucinations

Speech disorganization

Behavior disorganization

Negative symptoms

To meet the criteria for schizophrenia, patients must have had some disturbance for 6 months. During at least 1 month of this period, they must have two of the symptoms listed in the mnemonic; the other 5 months may include similar symptoms in attenuated form (i.e., prodromal or residual symptoms).

Substance Abuse

The same mnemonic, Tempted With Cognac, is used for criteria for any drug or alcohol dependence:

Tolerance (i.e., a need for increasing amounts of alcohol to achieve intoxication)

Withdrawal syndrome has occurred

Loss of Control of alcohol use (*encompasses the following five criteria*):
- Alcohol is often ingested in larger amounts than the patient intended.
- The patient has tried, unsuccessfully, to cut down.
- A great deal of time is spent in activities related to obtaining or recovering from the effects of alcohol.
- Important social, occupational, or recreational activities are given up or reduced because of alcohol use.
- Alcohol use is continued despite the patient's knowledge of significant physical or psychological problems caused by its use.

Three of the seven criteria listed above are required for diagnosis.

For alcohol dependence, the CAGE questionnaire is often used:

Have you felt you should Cut back on your drinking?

Has anybody Annoyed you with comments on your drinking?

Have you felt Guilty about your drinking?

Have you ever had an Eye-opener in the morning to get rid of a hangover?

Two or more affirmative answers indicate a high probability of alcohol dependence (Ewing 1984).

Anxiety Disorders

Panic Attack (four of 13).   With so many separate criteria to remember (13 total), trying to recall them with an acronym or phrase is not practical. My trick instead is to break the symptoms down into three clusters: (a) the heart, (b) breathlessness, and (c) fear. To remember them, I visualize a panicking patient clutching his chest (heart cluster), hyperventilating (breathlessness cluster), and shaking with fear (fear cluster). Finally, I imagine him screaming out, "Three-five-five! Three-five-five!"—presumably as a way of distracting himself from the panic attack. The numbers refer to the number of criteria in each cluster: The heart cluster has three criteria, and the other two clusters have five each.

I admit that this all sounds hokey, but believe me, you'll never forget the criteria if you do it!

HEART CLUSTER: THREE
I think of symptoms that often accompany a heart attack:

* Palpitations
* Chest pain
* Nausea

BREATHLESSNESS CLUSTER: FIVE
I think of symptoms associated with hyperventilation, which include dizziness, lightheadedness, tingling of the extremities or lips (parasthesias), and chills or hot flashes.

* Shortness of breath
* Choking sensation
* Dizziness
* Parasthesias
* Chills or hot flashes

FEAR CLUSTER: FIVE
I associate shaking and sweating with fear. To remember derealization, think of it as a way of psychologically escaping panic.

* Fear of dying
* Fear of going crazy
* Shaking
* Sweating
* Derealization or depersonalization

Aside from remembering the cluster names, remember the pattern 3-5-5 to keep from missing any of the 13 criteria. Your patient must have experienced four symptoms to meet the criteria for a full-scale panic attack.

Agoraphobia. I have no mnemonic for agoraphobia, because there are really only two criteria: a fear of being in places where escape might be difficult and efforts to avoid such places. See Chapter 23 for details.

Obsessive-Compulsive Disorder. The requirement for the diagnosis of OCD is the presence of obsessions, compulsions, or both to a degree that causes significant dysfunction. The definitions of obsessions and compulsions are easily learned and remembered (see Chapter 23), so a mnemonic is not necessary. Instead, I have chosen some of the most common symptoms seen in clinical practice; none of them is specifically required to be present by *DSM-IV.*

Washing and Straightening Make Clean Houses:

Washing

Straightening (ordering rituals)

Mental rituals (e.g., magical words, numbers)

Checking

Hoarding

Posttraumatic Stress Disorder. The PTSD patient Remembers Atrocious Nuclear Attacks.

Reexperiencing the trauma via intrusive memories, flashbacks, or nightmares (**one of which is required for diagnosis**)

Avoidance of stimuli associated with trauma and Numbing of general responsiveness (e.g., avoiding things associated with the trauma, amnesia for the trauma, restricted affect and activities, detachment, and foreshortened future; **one required for diagnosis**)

Symptoms of increased Arousal, such as insomnia, irritability, hypervigilance, startle response, and poor concentration (**two required for diagnosis**)

Generalized Anxiety Disorder (three of six). The first part of the diagnosis of GAD is easy: The patient has worried excessively about something for 6 months. The hard part is remembering the six anxiety symptoms, three of which must be present. The following mnemonic is based on the idea that Macbeth suffered GAD before and after killing King Duncan.

Macbeth Frets Constantly Regarding Illicit Sins:

Muscle tension

Fatigue

Concentration problems

Restlessness, feeling on edge

Irritability

Sleep problems

If this elaborate acronym isn't to your liking, an alternative is imagining what you would experience if you were constantly worrying about something or other. You'd have **insomnia**, leading to daytime **fatigue**. Fatigue in turn would cause **irritability** and **problems concentrating**, and constant worry would cause **muscle tension** and **restlessness**.

"Somatoform" Disorders*
Somatization Disorder
Recipe **4 pain**: **convert 2 stomachs** to **1 sex** (eight of eight symptoms, onset before age 30).

The diagnosis of somatization disorder requires a number of medically unexplained symptoms with onset before age 30. There must be four pain symptoms (4 pain), one conversion symptom (convert), two gastrointestinal symptoms (2 stomachs), and one sexual symptom (1 sex). This nonsensical mnemonic will lodge these criteria in your brain forever.

Bulimia Nervosa
Bulimics OverConsume Pastries (four of these):

Bingeing

Out-of-control feeling while eating

Concern with body shape

Purging

Anorexia Nervosa
Weight Fear Bothers Anorexics (four of these):

Weight below 85% of ideal body weight

---

*I use quotation marks because the eating disorders are not considered somatoform disorders by the *DSM-IV*. They are classified as such here for ease of memorization.

Fear of fat

Body image distortion

Amenorrhea

For both bulimia and anorexia, the patient must have all four criteria to merit the diagnosis.

Cognitive Disorders

Dementia.   (A memory impairment plus one of four BREW symptoms)

Memory **BREW**:

Memory impairment

Behavior disorganization (apraxia)

Recognition impairment (agnosia)

Executive functioning impairment

Word problems (aphasia)

Something is wrong with the "memory brew" of the patient with dementia. A gradual onset of a memory problem is required, but only one of the commonly associated symptoms (BREW) must be present. See Chapters 19 and 26 for further information on assessing these symptoms.

Delirium

Medical **FRAT** (all five of these):

Medical cause of cognitive impairment

Fluctuating course

Recent onset

Attention impairment

Thinking (cognitive) disturbance

Because delirium is caused by a medical illness, being part of the "medical fraternity" helps to diagnose it. To merit the diagnosis, all five criteria must be present. See Chapter 26 for details.

Attention-Deficit Hyperactivity Disorder.   There are 18 separate, though often redundant, criteria for ADHD, making memorization impossible for anyone without a photographic memory. As with panic disorder, I suggest breaking the symptoms into four broad categories, which can be remembered by the mnemonic **MOAT** (you'll need a MOAT around the classroom for the hyperactive child):

Movement excess (hyperactivity)

Organization problems (difficulty finishing tasks)

Attention problems

Talking impulsively

DSM-IV **criteria for ADHD**

A. Six of nine disorganization/inattention symptoms or six of nine impulsivity/hyperactivity symptoms must be present.
   Disorganization/inattention symptoms
   Organization problems
   - Can't organize tasks
   - Loses things needed for tasks
   - Problems finishing tasks
   Attention problems
   - Poor focus
   - Easily distracted
   - Doesn't listen
   - Forgets easily
   - Makes careless mistakes
   - Avoids tasks requiring concentration
   Impulsivity/hyperactivity symptoms
   Talking impulsively
   - Talks too much
   - Blurts out answers
   - Interrupts others
   - Can't play quietly
   Movement excess
   - Fidgets and squirms
   - Leaves seat
   - Displays restlessness
   - On the go
   - Can't wait for his turn

B. Some symptoms must have been present before age 7 years.
C. Symptoms occur in two or more settings, such as school (or work) and home.

Personality Disorders

Chapter 28 outlines a system for diagnosing personality disorders in general, including mnemonics for all ten of the personality disorders, which are not repeated here.

18

Interviewing for Diagnosis: The Art of Hypothesis Testing

Essential Concepts

- Use the free speech period for generating hypotheses.
- Investigate each hypothesis with screening and probing questions.
- Make graceful transitions to diagnostic questions throughout the interview.
- Use the PROS for "clean-up."

One might assume that the best way to come up with a diagnosis is to follow a two-step process:

1. Obtain all potentially relevant data about the patient.
2. Examine the data to determine which diagnosis fits best.

This strategy would work well if time were limitless. Because it isn't, clinicians have developed ways of determining in advance what is likely to be relevant data for a particular patient, thereby vastly increasing the efficiency of the diagnostic interview.

How do expert clinicians come up with diagnoses? A number of researchers have done observational studies to answer this question (Elstein et al. 1978; Kaplan 1995). They have found that experienced clinicians begin by carefully listening to the patient's initial complaint and asking open-ended questions. Based on this preliminary information, they generate a limited number of diagnostic hypotheses (the average being four) early in the interview, usually within the first 5 minutes. They then ask a number of closed-ended questions to test whether each hypothesis is true. This process is known as *pattern-matching*, in which the patient's pattern of symptoms is compared with the symptom pattern required for a diagnosis.

Another way to view this approach is to think of a "closed cone" of questions (Lipkin 1987). The initial questions are open ended and exploratory; they become more closed ended to pursue a specific diagnosis to an endpoint of verification or exclusion.

In accordance with these research-based conceptions, I suggest the following four stages for rapidly establishing diagnoses during the psychiatric interview.

FREE SPEECH PERIOD

In Chapter 3, I emphasize the value of giving the patient the opening word as a way of helping to create a therapeutic alliance, but it's also valuable for beginning the process of generating hypotheses. Generating diagnoses begins the moment you first see your patient and continues throughout the interview. It's important that your mind should be especially active during the first few minutes.

Keep the mnemonic "Depressed Patients Sound Anxious, So Claim Psychiatrists" in mind as you listen to your patient. Does she appear depressed or manic? Is she speaking coherently, and is her reality testing good? Does she seem anxious? Does she seem sharp or cognitively impaired? Is she beginning the interview complaining of numerous somatic symptoms? Does she have alcohol on her breath? Does she seem inappropriately angry or entitled? You will quickly be able to generate a mental list of likely diagnoses, which you should follow up on later in the interview with appropriate screening and probing questions.

SCREENING AND PROBING QUESTIONS

Once you've generated your short list of likely diagnoses, go on to test your hypotheses. Begin by asking a screening question that gets at the core feature of the disorder. Each disorder-specific chapter in Part III suggests one or more screening questions. For instance, a screening question for bipolar disorder (Chapter 21) is

> *Have you ever had a period of a week or so when you felt so happy and energetic that your friends said that you were talking too fast or that you were behaving differently and strangely?*

If the patient answers "yes," go right into the mnemonic for manic episodes (DIGFAST), and ask primarily closed-ended questions about each criterion. If the patient answers "no" and you are certain that he understood the question, you should conclude that bipolar disorder is unlikely and move onto another part of the interview.

Interviewing for diagnosis is an active, probing process in which you will often do as much talking as your patient. Is such an active style really more effective in eliciting diagnostic information than a quieter, listening style? Common sense dictates that it is, and the Maudsley Hospital researchers concluded that it is as well. In one of their papers examining techniques for eliciting factual information (Cox et al. 1981b), they found that a focused and directive style, in which interviewers used many probing questions and often requested detailed information, led to better data than a more passive style. The best data were obtained when interviewers used at least nine probing questions per symptom. Data were judged to be "better" when in addition to the mere mention of a symptom, such as depression, interviewers could obtain information about the frequency, duration, severity, context, and qualities of the symptom, all of which are extremely important for diagnostic decision making.

The concern remains that a directive style may elicit great factual data at the expense of shutting the patient down emotionally with too much questioning and not enough listening. Cox et al. (1981a) examined this issue and found that more directive interviewers actually elicited slightly more feelings than did interviewers with a less directive style.

TRANSITION GRACEFULLY TO DIAGNOSTIC QUESTIONS

 KEY POINT

Don't try to turn the diagnostic interview into a long checklist of diagnostic questions. This gives the interview a mechanical feeling and will diminish patient rapport. Instead, ask diagnostic questions at relevant points in the interview, using the transition skills you learned in Chapter 5. Much of Part III gives you tips for accomplishing such transitions; here are a few examples as a preview.

Illustrative Transitions to Diagnostic Areas

• Depression

> *With things so bad in your marriage, I wonder how it's been affecting your mood.*

- OCD

  You said you're often late. Are there rituals you do at home that make you late, like checking or cleaning things?

- Substance abuse

  Given all the stress you've been under, do you have a drink now and then to deal with it?

- Suicidality

  With things going so poorly in your life, I wonder if you've been debating whether it's worth it to go on?

- Borderline personality disorder

  Earlier you mentioned that your husband left you years ago; how do you normally deal with rejection?

- Psychosis

  You've been through so much stress lately—does it ever cause your mind to play tricks on you, so that you hear voices or have strange ideas?

PSYCHIATRIC REVIEW OF SYMPTOMS

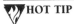 **HOT TIP**

It's not uncommon to forget to ask important questions during an interview, even if you use all the mnemonics in Chapter 17. The PROS is a helpful way to prevent this from happening. At some point toward the end of the interview, mentally review the *DSM-IV* mnemonic (**D**epressed **P**atients **S**ound **A**nxious, **S**o **C**laim **P**sychiatrists) and ask screening questions for any disorder that you haven't yet explored. This step resembles the survey approach that I decried earlier, but it's usually quite brief, because by this time you already will have covered the priority topics.

The PROS is usually best begun with an introduced transitional statement, such as

> *Now I'd like to switch gears a little and ask you about a bunch of different psychological symptoms some people have.*

Mental Status Examination

> **Essential Concepts**
>
> **Mnemonic for Elements of the Mental Status Examination:**
> **A**ll **B**orderline **S**ubjects **A**re **T**ough, **T**roubled **C**haracters
> - **A**ppearance
> - **B**ehavior
> - **S**peech
> - **A**ffect
> - **T**hought process (TP)
> - **T**hought content (TC)
> - **C**ognitive examination

Nothing in the psychiatric assessment is as misunderstood as the mental status examination (MSE). Two misconceptions are ubiquitous. The first is that the MSE takes place at the particular point in the interview when you test orientation and recall. In fact, the MSE occurs throughout the entire interview, during which you are constantly evaluating affect, concentration, memory, and insight. The second myth is that the MSE is identical to the Folstein Mini–Mental State Examination (MMSE). In fact, the Folstein MMSE is a specific screen for dementia. Increasingly, its use in the routine psychiatric interview is being questioned, but we'll talk more about that later.

The MSE is your evaluation of your patient's current state of cognitive and emotional functioning. Although most of the initial interview is specifically focused on your patient's past, doing an excellent MSE requires that you attend at the same time to his present. Here your "third ear" comes into play. How is your patient presenting himself? What is his TP like? How is he emoting? It will take you years to hone your powers of observation, and this is certainly the most interesting part of the diagnostic interview.

An MSE accomplishes two purposes. First, it helps make a diagnosis, especially in those cases in which historical data are unreliable or equivocal. A patient could send you an e-mail listing all of his depressive symptoms, but it requires direct observation—an MSE—to assess the degree of his anguish and his need for treatment. Second, the MSE allows you to create a vivid patient description for your records. Using this, you can more easily track your patient's progress from visit to visit, and you can give clinicians to whom you refer a more accurate sense of his condition.

ELEMENTS OF THE MENTAL STATUS EXAMINATION

The MSE has roughly seven components. This mnemonic will help you to remember them:

All Borderline Subjects Are Tough, Troubled Characters:

Appearance

Behavior

Speech

Affect

Thought process

Thought content

Cognitive examination

Appearance

How does your patient's appearance help you in your evaluation? At the extremes, a specific diagnosis might immediately suggest itself. For example, a disheveled man wearing bizarrely mismatched layers of clothes is schizophrenic until proven otherwise. Likewise, a flamboyant and seductively dressed woman with bright makeup who bounces into your office with energy to spare strongly suggests mania.

In usual clinical practice, however, these pathognomonic presentations are rare, and appearance provides more subtle, but no less useful, information. Qualities to note include

- Self-esteem: Does the patient care about his appearance? Compare the following two patient descriptions:

  The patient was a mildly overweight man with unruly black curly hair, dressed in ill-fitting baggy jeans and a T-shirt so tight that his stomach was visibly bulging above his belt.

> *The patient was a slim man who appeared younger than his 47 years, with fashionably cut short brown hair, an ironed button-down shirt, new jeans, and polished penny loafers.*

Both patients were diagnosed with depression, but they presented very differently and required different treatment plans.

- Personal statement: Does the appearance say something specific about your patient's interests, activities, or attitudes?

> *The patient came into the office dressed in a pressed electrician's uniform, with his name stitched over his breast pocket.*

> *She wore a T-shirt with the slogan, "Every day I'm forced to add one more name to the list of people who piss me off."*

- Memorable aspects: Describe whatever particularly strikes you about your patient. For example, if he is particularly attractive, note it, since degree of attractiveness is usually relevant to self-image. However, I have yet to see any report describe a patient as "unattractive," and I wouldn't recommend it, because it implies that you disliked him. Instead, describe the unattractive aspects.

> *This was a man of normal build who had a round, acne-covered face and was essentially bald, with the exception of small amounts of oily black hair on either side.*

Sometimes, a particular feature jumps out at you:

> *She had short curly brown hair, and her left eye was congenitally deviated toward the left, giving her a somewhat unsettling appearance.*

🐦 HOT TIP

The more vivid the notation, the better. I find it helpful to actually jot down a few descriptors at the beginning of the interview, during the free speech period.

Comment on height and build; hair color, style, and quality, including facial hair, if any; facial features, including eyes; clothes; movements; and any other prominent features of appearance, like tattoos or scars.

The following table (included in Appendix A as a pocket card) may appear to restate the obvious, but it's useful to me when I lack the right descriptive words.

Appearance terms

Aspect of appearance	Descriptors
Hair	Bald, thinning, close-cropped, short, long, shoulder-length, crew-cut, straight, curly, wavy, frizzy, braided, pony tail, pig tails, afro, relaxed, dread-locks, unevenly cut, stiff, greasy, dry, matted
Facial hair	Clean-shaven, neatly trimmed beard, long and scraggly beard, goatee, unshaven
Face	Attractive, nice-looking, pleasant, plain, pale, drawn, ruddy, flushed, bony, thin, broad, moon-shaped, red-nosed, thickly made-up
Eyes (gaze)	Good or poor eye contact, shifty, averted gaze, staring, fixated, dilated, downcast, forceful, intense, aggressive, piercing
Body	Thin, cachectic, lean, frail, underweight, normal build, muscular, husky, stocky, overweight, moderately obese, obese, morbidly obese, short, medium height, tall, tattooed arms
Movements	No abnormal movements, fidgety, bobbing knee, facial tic or twitch, lip smacking, lip puckering, tremulous, jittery, restless, wringing hands, motionless, rigid, limp, stiff, slumped
Clothes	Casually dressed, neat, appropriate, professional, immaculate, fashionable, sloppy, ill-fitting, out-dated, flamboyant, sexually provocative, soiled, dirty, tight, loose, slogans on clothes

Behavior and Attitude

How did your patient behave toward you when you first met her? Was she friendly and cooperative, or did she seem indifferent and apathetic? Did she sit right down and face you, or was she agitated, pacing around the room and talking rapidly without really attending to your questions? The context of the interview may also be important to making sense of the behavior. Was it a scheduled evaluation interview or did it take place in an emergency room?

Descriptors of attitude are similar to descriptors of affect (see the table on page 124), but the emphasis is on words that describe a relationship toward someone. Often, a sentence of description is important. Here are some examples:

> *He presented himself as someone who was very anxious to tell his story and to gain relief from his symptoms. He had an attitude of submissive respect, saying things like, "Do you think you can help me, doctor? What do you think I have?"*

> *She presented as indifferent and apathetic. Her general attitude was that this was just the latest in a long string of unhelpful interviews.*

Often, your patient's attitude toward you will change over the course of the interview.

> *He was initially reluctant to answer questions and seemed irritable. Over the course of the interview, he became more self-revealing and tearful.*

Speech

Description of speech has great overlap with description of TP, since we can only know our patients' thoughts through speech. Qualities of speech to consider include

- Rate: Does he speak rapidly or slowly? Rapid or "pressured" speech is usually a buzzword for manic speech, but you need to be careful not to overpathologize. Rapid speech can signal anxiety or even be the normal speech pattern. We all know people who speak very rapidly but are not manic.
- Volume: Patients who speak loudly may be manic, irritable, or anxious. Very low volume may signal depression or shyness. Again, loud or quiet speech may also be a nonpathologic variant of normal.
- Latency of response: Normally, when you are asked a question, you'll think for a fraction of a second before responding. This is the normal latency of response. Manic patients may respond so quickly that they seem to jump onto the last few words of your questions. Depressed or psychotic patients may show an increased latency of response, waiting several seconds before answering simple questions.

- General quality: Does your patient speak thoughtfully and in an articulate manner, or does she ramble in a vague and disconnected way, making her hard to follow? These terms are discussed in more detail in Chapter 25, in the section on disorders of TP.

Speech terms

Normal
Thoughtful
Articulate
Intelligent
Rapid
Staccato
Pressured
Rambling
Continuous
Loud
Soft
Barely audible
Slow
Halting

Affect and Mood

Traditional teaching distinguishes mood from affect, with *mood* defined as a patient's subjective report of how he feels, and *affect* defined as your own impression of his emotional state. Although many clinicians do not make this distinction in clinical work, you should become familiar with it, because it is widely used.

Like observation of appearance and behavior, accurate observation of affect is a skill that takes years to master. While the overall emotional flavor is usually obvious, the gradations and subtleties are not, and assessing degree of affect can be vitally important for such things as determining imminence of SI or predicting the likelihood of aggressive acting out.

Often, you won't have to explicitly ask your patient how he's been feeling, because he'll report it spontaneously. However, what do you do when your patient is vague about his emotions or is reluctant to reveal himself?

The obvious (and easiest) approach is to come right out and ask.

> *How do you feel right now? How has your mood been over the past few days?*

If the patient answers with a vague term, follow up with questions aimed at giving a more refined name to the affect, a name on which you both can agree but which you have not "fed" the patient.

CLINICAL VIGNETTE

> I: *How have you been feeling over the past few days?*
>
> P: *Not so great.*
>
> I: *Hmmm. Not so great. Can you give that feeling a name?*
>
> P: *Just . . . really lousy.*
>
> I: *I mean an emotion word, like sad, nervous, angry, and so on.*
>
> P: *Sad, I guess.*

One particularly difficult situation is when your patient says he feels "up and down" or that he has "mood swings." Suddenly you are faced with a huge diagnostic differential. Does the patient have bipolar disorder? Cyclothymia? Does he have depression with mood reactivity? Does he have a personality disorder? An anxiety disorder? A substance abuse disorder? All of these are compatible with an up-and-down mood.

Your questioning strategy should be based on trying to locate an enduring, persistent mood beneath the variations. Or, if there is true mood instability, you should determine whether the lows meet criteria for major depression and the highs satisfy criteria for mania. I'll have more to say about these issues in Chapters 21 and 22, but here's an example of a strategy that usually works well:

CLINICAL VIGNETTE

> I: *How have you been feeling over the past few days?*
>
> P: *(Shaking head, looking at interviewer intensely.) Totally up and down.*
>
> I: *Tell me about the downs first. When you say "down," do you mean sad or depressed, or something else?*

P: *Really depressed.*

I: *Do you feel depressed nearly every day?*

P: *Sometimes I get really happy.*

I: *I want to talk about the happy times, too, in a second. To focus on the down times, do you have depressed periods nearly every day?*

P: *Yes.*

I: *Is your concentration affected during those depressed periods?*

[The interviewer goes through the neurovegetative symptoms (NVSs) of depression and determines that the patient meets criteria for a major depressive episode.]

I: *Now, tell me more about the really happy times you've been having. What do you mean by "ups"?*

P: *Feeling great, feeling on top of the world.*

I: *Okay. Do you really feel great nearly every day?*

P: *No, not every day, but sometimes I do.*

I: *Over the past 2 weeks, how many days would you say you felt really great?*

P: *Oh, a couple. My parents gave me a car for graduation. I was so happy.*

I: *How long did that happy mood last?*

P: *Couple of days.*

I: *Then how did you feel?*

P: *Down, as usual.*

The eventual diagnosis was major depression, because the patient's pervasive mood had been depression, with a number of the required NVSs. The "ups" turned out to be brief reprieves from the persistent depressed mood.

The following table (included as a pocket card in Appendix A) is a useful reference while you're writing up the MSE. Use it to enrich your emotional vocabulary, so that you don't get in the habit of using a single word to describe all patients with a particular kind of affect.

Affect terms

Affect	Terms
Normal	Appropriate, calm, pleasant, relaxed, normal, friendly, comfortable, unremarkable
Happy	Cheerful, bright, peppy, content, self-satisfied, silly, giggly, grandiose, euphoric, elated, exalted
Sad	Sad, gloomy, sullen, depressed, pessimistic, morose, hopeless, discouraged
Anxious	Anxious, worried, tense, nervous, apprehensive, frightened, terrified, bewildered, paranoid
Angry	Angry, irritable, disdainful, bitter, arrogant, defensive, sarcastic, annoyed, furious, enraged, hostile
Indifferent	Indifferent, shallow, superficial, cool, distant, apathetic, aloof, dull, vacant, affectless, uninterested, cynical

Qualities of Affect

Four qualities of affect are commonly taught, but, as with the distinction between mood and affect, the usefulness of these distinctions is controversial. My opinion is that there is too much hair-splitting in academic psychiatry, and that clinical work would be simpler and just as effective without worrying about the following distinctions. Nonetheless, many would disagree, and you should at least become familiar with the terms, whether or not you use them.

1. *Stability of affect:* This refers to a continuum from *stable* affect (generally defined as normal) to *labile* affect (generally abnormal). Marked lability of affect (e.g., when a patient alternates between giggling and uncontrollable sobbing) is usually a marker of either mania or acute psychosis, but it may also be seen in dementia and other neuropsychiatric syndromes.

2. *Appropriateness:* A patient who laughs uncontrollably while talking about her mother's death is exhibiting inappropriate affect, and this is useful to record. Inappropriate affect is often seen in psychosis or mania. Don't overpathologize, however; many intact people smile a bit when talking about sad things. This may reflect a defense mechanism such as denial, rather than psychosis.

3. *Range of affect:* Mentally healthy humans exhibit a full range of affect. At some moments they feel happy, at other moments annoyed, and at others sad. Depressed patients are

said to exhibit *constricted* affect, and schizophrenics are often said to exhibit *flat* affect. The problem, of course, is that many normal people exhibit a narrow range of affect. This may be especially true during a psychiatric interview, because patients may not feel emotionally safe exposing themselves to a stranger. Thus, the diagnostic specificity of a limited range of affect is suspect and should not be overinterpreted.

4. *Intensity of affect*: Intensity is often hard to distinguish from range of affect, and like range, the diagnostic specificity is unknown. The usual jargon describes three grades: intense, flat, and blunted. *Flat* and *blunted* are usually reserved for descriptions of severely depressed patients or patients with negative symptoms of schizophrenia. *Intense* is often used for manic or histrionic patients, but remember that many completely healthy people come across as passionate or intense.

Thought Process

TP refers to the flow of thought (coherent vs. incoherent) and is covered in detail in Chapter 25.

Thought Content

TC refers to unusual or dangerous ideas and includes SI and homicidal ideation (HI) (see Chapter 20); psychotic ideation, such as delusions and hallucinations (see Chapter 25); and any significant themes that came up during the interview and relate to the psychiatric diagnosis.

Cognitive Examination

What are the essential components of the screening cognitive examination? Unfortunately, there is no general agreement on this issue, and many clinicians argue that much of what is commonly taught as essential to the cognitive examination is of questionable use (Rapp 1979). For example, most training programs continue to teach the serial sevens subtraction test (SSST) of attention, even though studies have demonstrated that it has little validity in separating demented patients from normal patients. (See the section on Attention and Concentration for a more complete discussion.) Many of the other commonly taught elements of the cognitive examination are equally suspect, including the digit span test, abstractions, similarities, proverbs, and judgment questions (Keller and Manschreck 1989).

I focus here on what is truly useful in helping you to differentiate between normal and impaired cognition. You should be aware, however, that this is a screening approach only. Specialized tests of cognitive abilities, usually conducted by a neuropsychologist, should be done if your screening indicates a potential problem.

▼ **Caveat:** A number of studies have shown that low educational attainment correlates with poor performance on cognitive testing in the absence of dementia or other organic impairments (Ainslie and Murden 1993; Anthony et al. 1982; Murden et al. 1991). Most studies have defined *poorly educated* as 8 or fewer years of education, that is, no high school. The implication for clinicians is that you should ask about educational level before testing and be cautious about overinterpreting cognitive abnormalities in poorly educated patients.

The elements of cognition that you should assess include

- Level of awareness or wakefulness
- Attention and concentration
- Memory
- Judgment
- Insight

Perception is important too, of course, but its assessment is discussed in Chapter 25.

Level of Awareness or Wakefulness

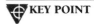 **KEY POINT**

The continuum of wakefulness ranges from comatose to fully alert. Determining the level of wakefulness is important for two reasons. First, it will clue you in to certain diagnoses, such as benzodiazepine or alcohol abuse in the drowsy patient or mania or stimulant abuse in the hyperalert patient. Second, it will give you guidance in how to proceed with the rest of the cognitive examination. For example, a full cognitive examination is not valid in a patient who is nodding off throughout the interview.

The assessment of wakefulness is easy enough. Your first 10 seconds of contact with a patient will tell you whether he is alert enough to greet you appropriately and tell you his name.

If he seems sleepy, you have at your disposal an entire lexicon for describing degrees of sleepiness: sleepy, drowsy, lethargic, somnolent, stuporous, obtunded, and comatose. Because there are no generally agreed-on definitions of most of these terms, it's best to describe the degree of sleepiness in plain English. Thus, instead of "stuporous," say,

> *The patient was sleepy, and could only be awakened by my calling his name loudly and shaking his shoulder.*

Instead of "drowsy," say,

> *The patient yawned frequently during the interview but attended well to all questions.*

> *The patient nodded off frequently and had difficulty resuming his train of thought.*

These descriptions help the reader of your assessment to draw conclusions regarding the reliability of the rest of the MSE.

Attention and Concentration.   You want to assess whether your patient can sustain attention over a period of time. The continuum of attention runs from attentive and focused at one end to confused and distractible at the other.

Most training programs teach two tests for assessing attention: the digit span test and the SSST. In the digit span test, the patient is given five to seven numbers and asked to repeat them forward and backward; in the SSST, the patient is asked to subtract seven from 100 and to continue counting back by sevens until told to stop. Both of these tasks intuitively seem like reasonable tests of attention; unfortunately, research studies have not endorsed them.

In one study (Smith 1967), the SSST was given to 132 normal adults aged 18 to 63, all of whom were fully employed and the majority of whom had at least 16 years of education. The professions represented included psychiatry, psychology, neurology, and pediatrics. Only 42% of these subjects had errorless performance on the SSST. Fully 31 of the subjects made between three and 12 errors, and 14 either gave stereotyped responses (supposedly consistent with frontal lobe disease) or totally abandoned the task. In another study (Milstein et al. 1972), 325 hospitalized psychiatric patients were given the SSST. No difference in performance between patients and 50 normal control subjects appeared, and there was no association between poor performance on the test and the presence of organic cognitive impairments. With regard to the digit span test, Crook et al.

(1980) found no difference in seven-digit recall among 60 elderly patients who had memory impairment and 44 elderly people who were normal.

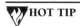**HOT TIP**

The best way to assess attention and concentration is simply to talk to your patient and observe how she thinks. Is she able to concentrate on your questions? Can she maintain a train of thought as she answers you? If the answer to these questions is "yes," your patient's attention is intact.

Memory.   You should assess both short-term memory (memory of things learned a few minutes to a few days ago) and long-term memory (memory of things learned longer than a few days ago). Studies have documented that the most clinically valid tests of these are (a) orientation, (b) three-object recall, (c) recall of remote personal events, and (d) recall of general cultural information (Keller and Manschrek 1989).

ORIENTATION

Orientation to person, place, and time is often thought to be a specific test of delirium or confusion, but it is actually a test of memory. One's name, one's location, and the date are all pieces of information that must be learned and retained. Whereas one's name is invariant, and therefore is encoded in long-term memory, both the date and the place change often, offering ideal ways to test whether people are capable of retaining new information.

Because asking people where they are and what the date is can feel awkward, here are some ways to transition into these questions smoothly. You can introduce all your memory questions with a statement such as

> I'd like to change gears here and ask you a few questions to test your memory.

Often, you can make a smooth transition from some information you just obtained:

> (The patient just told you her father had Alzheimer's disease.) Speaking of that, how has your memory been? I'd like to ask you some questions to test your memory.
>
> (The patient said his concentration has been poor while he's been depressed.) Speaking of concentration,

I'd like to ask a few questions to test how your memory and concentration are doing now.

Once you've introduced the need to assess memory, you can go into your orientation questions with a question such as

Do you keep track of time pretty well?

Regardless of the response, you can follow up with

For example, would you be able to tell me today's date?

 HOT TIP

If your patient is taking a while and struggling to remember, a time-saving tip is to ask about specific components, going from easiest to hardest.

What year is it? What month? What day of the week? And what's the date?

▼ **Caveat:** Don't overinterpret an inaccurate date. Many cognitively intact people don't keep close track of the date. To prove this to yourself, ask yourself what the date is today. If you're off by a day, you're normal. Thus, in recording your MSE, rather than writing "patient was not oriented to date," record instead what the patient said. Assuming, for example, that the true date is Wednesday, August 19, 1998, there is a world of difference between the patient who says "Wednesday, August 18, 1998," and the patient who answers, "sometime in '64."

THREE-OBJECT RECALL

Recall of three objects after at least 2 minutes has been shown to be a useful test in diagnosing cognitive impairments (Hinton and Withers 1971). Say to your patient,

Repeat the following three words: ball, chair, purple.

Make sure your patient can repeat them correctly before moving on. You must be satisfied that your patient has correctly registered all three of the words, because otherwise your test of memory will not be valid. Some elderly patients may have difficulty repeating the words because of a hearing problem. (One of my hard-of-hearing patients repeated the words as "pall, share, gurgle.") In such cases, repeat the words more loudly until they have registered. You may encounter a similar problem if English is not your patient's first language. Of course, if your patient is extremely demented or confused, she will not be able to repeat the words for that reason. However, patients with such severe cognitive impairment will have already been diagnosed because of difficulties in answering basic informational questions early in the interview.

Once you are satisfied that your patient has registered all three words, say,

> *Now I want you to remember those three words, because I'm going to ask you to repeat them in a couple of minutes.*

In the meantime, ask your patient general knowledge questions (see below) about general cultural and personal information. Then ask him to repeat the three words.

If your patient has trouble, use the following hints:

> *One of them is something you can play with.*
>
> *One is a piece of furniture.*
>
> *One is a color.*

Cognitively normal people usually remember all three words, and if they forget one they will remember it after your hint. Performance any worse than that indicates a possible problem in short-term memory.

GENERAL CULTURAL KNOWLEDGE
Certain items of cultural and historical information have been so widely taught that you can assume any American with at least a high school education has learned them. Inability to recall at least half of these items is presumptive evidence of long-term memory impairment.

 HOT TIP

The traditional task is to name the last five presidents, although there's no evidence that there is anything magical about the number five. In practice, cognitively intact patients commonly have problems remembering that Carter came before Reagan and that Ford came before Carter. Therefore, I recommend asking about the last three presidents.

- Last three presidents: Begin with

    Who is the current president?

  Then

    Who was president before Clinton?

    Who was before Bush?

- Other famous figures: I ask about people who are so enduringly famous that the average person can't get through a typical month without hearing a reference to them.

    Who was _____? What was he/she famous for?

  Here are a few of these famous people, along with what a cognitively intact person should be able to tell you about them:

  George Washington, first president

  Abraham Lincoln, freed the slaves

  Martin Luther King, Jr., civil rights leader

  Princess Diana, British princess killed in car accident

  William Shakespeare, writer

  Christopher Columbus, discovered America

- Famous dates: In asking these questions, you should not expect a precisely correct response, but rather a response that names a year in the ballpark.

    When did World War II happen? (Any time in the 1930s or 1940s is adequate.)

    When was JFK assassinated? (Sometime in the 1960s.)

- Lists of information: A highly sensitive approach to screening for dementia is the Set test, first described in 1973 (Isaacs and Kennie 1973). The procedure is to ask your patient to name as many items (up to ten) as he can recall in each of four categories: colors, animals, fruits, and towns. Out of a maximum of 40, a score of 25 or above excluded the diagnosis of dementia in the original study.

PERSONAL KNOWLEDGE

Personal knowledge includes aspects of current life as well as memory of remote personal events. Cognitively intact patients should be able to tell you

- Current address and phone number
- Names and ages of spouse, siblings, and children
- Spouse's birthday, wedding anniversary, and date and place of marriage (if married)
- Parents' names and birthdays (primarily for younger patients who are not married)

 HOT TIP

How do you know if the patient's answer is accurate? Address, phone number, and spouse's name are often on the chart's registration sheet. You can check the other information by calling a family member. Generally, however, patients do not blatantly confabulate, alcoholic dementia being the major exception to this, and you can often get a sense of cognitive status without resorting to time-consuming phone calls.

Intelligence.   As with concentration, you can get a general idea of level of intelligence via the rest of the interview. Think of intelligence as the ability to manipulate information. High levels of educational and job attainment usually correlate with high intelligence.

 HOT TIP

For a quick and dirty measure of IQ, you can give the easy-to-remember Wilson Rapid Approximate Intelligence Test (Wilson 1967). Start with 2×48 as a screening test. If the patient can calculate this, she's very unlikely to be in the borderline or retarded range, and you can end the testing. Patients who can't calculate 2×24 are likely to meet IQ criteria for mental retardation and should definitely be referred for formal neuropsychological testing. The usual caveat regarding educational level applies: You should only give this test to patients who have completed high school.

Wilson Rapid Approximate Intelligence Test

Intelligence	Best effort	IQ (rough estimate)
Retarded	2×6	<70
Borderline	2×24	70–80
Dull normal	2×48	80–90
Average	2×384	90–110
Bright normal	$2 \times 1,536$	110–120
Superior	$2 \times 3,072$	120–130

Insight

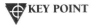

KEY POINT

Although the term *insight* has many layers of meaning, for the purposes of the evaluation interview you are most interested in whether your patient knows that he has an illness and has some realistic conception of its causes and possible treatments.

Sometimes a patient's lack of insight is blatant. Such is the case with many manic and schizophrenic patients, who may be absolutely convinced of the veracity of their delusions. Documenting poor insight in such cases is easy, but in many cases you have to probe for degree of insight by asking, often toward the end of the interview,

> *So, why do you think you've been having these problems?*
>
> *What do you think needs to happen for your life to improve?*

Insightful patients will be able to identify some psychosocial stressors related to their disorder (either as cause or effect). Patients with poor insight might respond with phrases such as

> *I don't know. You're the doctor.*
>
> *People need to stop hassling me. (A paranoid patient.)*

Whereas complete lack of insight is often seen in psychotic disorders or dementia, poor insight might point you at a diagnosis of a character disorder or low intelligence.

Judgment.   The standard question for testing judgment is by now widely recognized as unhelpful in assessing the sort of judgment in which clinicians are interested:

> *If you found a stamped and addressed envelope laying on the sidewalk, what would you do?*

Instead, you should assess judgment based on the material gathered throughout the interview. Did your patient decide to seek help when she felt depressed? Did she apply for unemployment benefits when she lost her job? These show good judgment. Did she decide that the best treatment for her depression was to go on a cocaine binge? This shows poor judgment.

Often, students lump tests of abstraction with tests of judgment. These include the interpretation of proverbs and the recognition of similarities. These tests show very low interrater reliability (Andreason et al. 1974), they show no demonstrated usefulness in the diagnosis of organic problems, and good performance is highly correlated with intelligence (Keller and Manschreck 1989), which is generally not what the tests are supposed to be testing.

SHOULD YOU USE THE FOLSTEIN MINI–MENTAL STATE EXAMINATION?

The Folstein MMSE (Folstein et al. 1975) contains 11 categories of scored questions. The maximum possible score is 30, and scores below 30 may indicate cognitive impairment, with the precise cutoff point varying by age and education. The sensitivity of the test is high—you're unlikely to miss cases of dementia—but the specificity is low, meaning that many patients who are cognitively normal will be misclassified as demented. This happened in 17% of patients in one study (Anthony et al. 1982).

Whether the MMSE should be used in all psychiatric evaluations is a matter of great controversy. Proponents argue that its high sensitivity makes it essential, and that a numerical measure of cognitive functioning is a great help in tracking the course of dementia. Opponents argue that the test's positive predictive value is unacceptably low, and that it is less sensitive and specific than clinical judgment that is based on the results of the entire interview (Harwood et al. 1997; Tangalos et al. 1996).

The MMSE is most useful for clinicians with little training in the psychiatric interview who need a standardized format for asking a series of questions. It is less useful for mental health clinicians, since we can skillfully ascertain cognitive functioning from the interview as a whole and can target particular questions to assess specific areas of possible impairment. In addition, the MMSE includes one test that has been found to be invalid for evaluating cognitive impairment (SSST) and does *not* include other questions that are very important in assessing for dementia, such as questions about personal and general knowledge.

Notwithstanding the many limitations of the MMSE, it is used so widely in a variety of clinical settings that you should become familiar with it. (The test is reproduced in Appendix A, along with age- and education-adjusted norms.)

20 ▼ Assessing Suicidal and Homicidal Ideation

> **Essential Concepts**
>
> **Suicidal Ideation**
> - Learn the **SAD PERSONS** risk factors for suicide.
> - Assess passive suicidality.
> - Assess active suicidality.
> - Assess imminent plan.
>
> **Homicidal Ideation**
> - Learn the risk factors for homicide.
> - Ask about HI.
> - Know your Tarasoff duties.

We cannot tear out a single page from our life, but we can throw the whole book into the fire.

George Sand

RISK FACTORS FOR SUICIDE

The reason an assessment of suicidality is necessary in every diagnostic interview is obvious enough: We hope to prevent suicide. Unfortunately, the mental health field has not yet devised tools that allow prediction of suicidal behavior in a particular patient. On the other hand, researchers have discovered a number of factors that increase the statistical risk for suicide. It is important to be aware of these risk factors as you interview any potentially suicidal patient.

In evaluating suicidality during the initial interview, you have two goals. The first and most important is to assess whether an immediate risk of a suicide attempt exists. Your second goal is to determine current or past suicidality to help you formulate an accurate *DSM-IV* diagnosis. You can achieve both of these goals with the same line of questioning.

Before reviewing the types of questions to ask, you should be familiar with the risk factors for suicide. An excellent mnemonic for the major risk factors is "SAD PERSONS" (reproduced as a pocket card in Appendix A), devised by Patterson et al. (1983).

Mnemonic: **SAD PERSONS** (risk factors for suicide)

Sex: Woman are more likely to attempt suicide; men are more likely to succeed.

Age: Age falls into a bimodal distribution, with teenagers and the elderly at highest risk.

Depression: Fifteen percent of depressives die by suicide.

Previous attempt: Ten percent of those who have previously attempted suicide die by suicide.

Ethanol abuse: Fifteen percent of alcoholics commit suicide.

Rational thinking loss: Psychosis is a risk factor, and 10% of chronic schizophrenics die by suicide.

Social supports are lacking.

Organized plan: A well-formulated suicide plan is a red flag.

No spouse: Being divorced, separated, or widowed is a risk factor; having responsibility for children is an important statistical protector against suicide.

Sickness: Chronic illness is a risk factor.

Although useful for determining a patient's long-term risk for committing suicide, these risk factors are less useful for assessing imminent risk, and imminent risk is the most important factor to assess during a diagnostic interview. One study helpful in identifying risk factors for short-term risk is the National Institute of Mental Health Collaborative Depression Clinical Study (Clark and Fawcett 1992). Researchers followed 954 patients with major affective disorders and found that clinical features associated with early suicide (i.e., within 1 year of assessment) included

- Anxiety
- Panic attacks
- Anhedonia
- Alcohol abuse

Clinical factors associated with a later attempt (at 5 years) included

- High levels of hopelessness
- SI
- History of suicide attempts

ASSESSING SUICIDAL IDEATION: INTERVIEW STRATEGIES

KEY POINT

Suicidality can be a difficult topic to broach, but you must ask about it in every diagnostic interview. Patients are rarely angry or embarrassed about suicidality questions. A majority of depressed patients have at least passing suicidal thoughts from time to time (Winokur 1981), and many patients are relieved when they are asked about suicidality, because it allows them to reveal the true depth of their depression. If they really have not thought about suicide, they will say something like, "Oh no, I could never do anything like that," and will tell you why not.

Another common disincentive to asking about suicidality is the interviewer's fear of a positive response. You may feel a sense of panic when first confronted with a suicidal patient, but with experience you will realize that there are degrees of suicidality, and that not all suicidal patients require urgent hospitalization.

The suicidality issue can be approached in a number of ways. The direct approach can be perfectly acceptable. For example, as part of your evaluation of the SIGECAPS of depression, you can say,

> *Have you felt suicidal?*
>
> *Have you had thoughts of wanting to hurt yourself?*

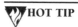**HOT TIP**

In some situations, however, this approach may feel jarring to the patient, and a smooth transition may be better:

> *Sometimes when people feel depressed, they think that they'd be better off dead. Has that thought crossed your mind at all?*
>
> *Considering all the things you've told me, have you felt so bad that it seems that life is not worth living?*

These are both normalizing questions that inquire about "passive" SI. If you get a "yes," you should ask about active SI.

Have you thought about suicide?

What sorts of ways have you thought about to hurt yourself? (Phrased as a behavior expectation.)

Many people with mild to moderate depression endorse passive SI but deny having thought of actually taking some action to harm themselves. This an important clinical distinction, and you can generally breathe easier if your patient's SI has never gotten beyond the passive stage. If, however, your patient admits to active SI, you'll need to ask an additional series of questions. You want to find out how elaborate and how realistic the suicide plan is.

Have you thought about cutting yourself?

Taking an overdose?

Jumping from the window?

Shooting yourself?

Hanging yourself?

Don't worry that you are putting ideas into their heads. By inquiring specifically about common suicidal behaviors, you are giving patients permission to be truthful and communicating that you're familiar with this difficult topic and won't be put off by a positive answer.

How close have you come to actually hurting yourself?

Have you planned it out in your mind?

Have you acquired any of the things you would need to do something?

Here, you're asking about the presence of a plan and getting a sense of how close the patient has come to carrying out his plan.

Have you actually had the pills in your hand with a glass of water in front of you?

Have you put the pills in your mouth?

What prevented you from actually swallowing them?

This continues specific questioning. The same line of questioning can be used with any other method of suicide the patient may have been fantasizing about.

Do you have a gun in the house?

Do you have access to a rope?

Do you have pills at home?

You should assess how realistic the plan communicated by your patient is. If a patient says he wants to shoot himself, this sounds quite serious, but does he own a gun? If not, does he have access to a friend or relative's gun? Has he located a shop at which he plans to buy a gun?

Have you written a suicide note?

Have you done anything to put your affairs in order in preparation for your death?

Arrangements such as these are particularly ominous indicators of an imminent suicide attempt.

Are you feeling suicidal right now? Do you have any specific plan to hurt yourself?

Here, you are asking about the immediacy of the intention, so that you can determine the necessity for hospitalization or other urgent intervention.

What has kept you from killing yourself?

This is a very useful topic to introduce. Many desperate patients remain adamantly opposed to suicide for specific reasons, often because they have dependent children or on religious grounds. If you can identify compelling factors that are keeping your patient in the land of the living, reinforce them.

If you were to feel more suicidal over the next few days, do you think you could promise to pick up the phone and talk to someone before actually hurting yourself, or would you be in so much pain that you wouldn't want to ask for help?

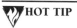**HOT TIP**

Here you are trying to discover whether the patient is able to "contract for safety." The whole notion of a safety contract is controversial, and such a contract can certainly provide a false sense of reassurance to the clinician. My feeling is that safety contracts at least do no harm, and that they probably have saved lives, because they offer a concrete plan to someone who may be experiencing too much turmoil to think clearly. A good safety contract includes names and numbers of people the patient agrees to contact and a way for her to contact you or your coverage.

ASSESSING HOMICIDAL IDEATION

 KEY POINT

Although I have combined the assessment of HI with the assessment of SI, the two are very different creatures. You should assess SI in every patient you interview, but you will ask about HI only in patients you feel are at risk of becoming homicidal. This includes patients in groups that have been identified by researchers as at high risk for homicide (Asnis et al. 1994; Tardiff 1992), such as those who are paranoid, antisocial, or substance abusers or who tell you they are angry at someone in particular.

HI is not the easiest topic to broach during the interview. Interview techniques (see Chapter 4) such as normalization and reduction of guilt are helpful. Once you have introduced the topic, your strategy should be to determine exactly who is the target of the HI and then to assess the seriousness of the ideation. This process is analogous to the assessment of SI, in which you must locate the ideation on a continuum from passive to active to a specific and imminent plan.

CLINICAL VIGNETTE

A 35-year-old woman was admitted to the hospital with the delusion that her mother had been replaced by an impostor who was attempting to take possession of the family home. Knowing that paranoia is a risk factor for HI, the interviewer decided to assess this possibility.

> I: *How do you feel about this woman? (Referring to the "impostor" mother.)*
>
> P: *How would you feel? She's taking away all that is mine.*
>
> I: *I'd be very angry.*

P: *There you go. I'm being wronged.*

I: *I imagine someone in your situation would go to great lengths to prevent this from happening. (Using normalization.)*

P: *I'd say so.*

I: *Even to the extent of wanting to do away with that person?*

P: *She's raping my heritage. Death would be too good for her.*

I: *It sounds like you'd be happy if she were dead.*

P: *(Looking at interviewer incredulously.) Of course I would.*

(At this point, the interviewer has established passive HI; he must now assess whether there is active HI.)

I: *Have you thought about killing her yourself?*

P: *I wish I could. But there are too many others just like her. If I killed her, they would know who did it, and they'd come after me.*

I: *So you haven't come up with a plan for killing her?*

P: *Plenty of plans, but where will that get me? I told you, I can't do it.*

I: *What sorts of plans?*

P: *The best way would be to cremate her in the house that she wants so much.*

I: *You mean set fire to the house?*

P: *It would break my heart to lose the house, but that may be necessary.*

The interviewer concluded that the patient was at high risk of following through on her plan to torch her mother's house as a homicide attempt.

___

This vignette brings up the important issue of what you should do when a patient expresses HI. The Tarasoff decision of 1976 provides guidelines for mental health professionals

(Felthous 1991). In essence, you have a responsibility to protect the potential victim. This generally entails informing both the potential victim and the police.

If you do decide to issue a Tarasoff warning, informing your patient of your intentions is a good idea. In such cases, a straightforward approach works best.

> *The law requires me to do what I can to keep this person safe. That means I'm going to try to call him and also call the police.*

You may worry that telling the patient about your intentions will harm the therapeutic alliance. However, according to the only study that actually looked at this issue, in most cases issuing a warning had either a minimal negative or a positive effect on the alliance (Binder and McNiel 1996).

Assessing Mood Disorders I: Depressive Disorders

Essential Concepts

Screening Questions
- Are you depressed?
- Have you ever gone through a 2-year (for the diagnosis of dysthymia) period of feeling sad most of the time?

Mnemonic: **SIGECAPS**

Recommended time: 1 minute if screen is negative; 5 minutes if screen is positive

Diagnosis of the different types of depressive disorders begins with diagnosis of a major depressive episode. Once you become expert at assessing the presence of the NVSs of depression, you will be able to diagnose quickly major depression, atypical depression, seasonal affective disorder (SAD), and dysthymic disorder.

KEY POINT

It is equally important that you know when *not* to diagnose a depressive disorder. Major depression tends to get a disproportionate amount of attention in mental health education, partly because it is genuinely common and partly because we are so good at treating it. Nonetheless, you do a disservice to a patient by diagnosing him with major depression if instead he has an adjustment disorder with depressed mood and would benefit more from brief psychotherapy than from medication.

MAJOR DEPRESSIVE EPISODE

DSM-IV Criteria
Five or more of the following symptoms have been present for at least 2 weeks; at least one of the symptoms is either (a) depressed mood or (b) loss of interest or pleasure.

- Depressed mood most of the day, nearly every day
- Markedly diminished interest or pleasure in all, or almost all, activities
- Decrease in appetite or significant weight loss
- Insomnia or hypersomnia
- Psychomotor agitation or retardation
- Fatigue or loss of energy
- Feelings of worthlessness or excessive or inappropriate guilt
- Diminished concentration or indecisiveness
- Thoughts of death or SI

Mnemonic: SIGECAPS

Mnemonic: SIGECAPS

A useful mnemonic to guide your questioning of the NVSs of depression is SIGECAPS. It was devised by Dr. Carey Gross at Massachusetts General Hospital and refers to what one might write on a prescription sheet for a depressed, anergic patient: **SIG**: Energy **CAP**sules. Each letter refers to one of the major diagnostic criteria for major depressive disorder:

Sleep disorder (either increased or decreased)*

Interest deficit (anhedonia)

Guilt (worthlessness,* hopelessness,* regret)

Energy deficit*

Concentration deficit*

Appetite disorder (either decreased or increased)*

Psychomotor retardation or agitation

Suicidality

For dysthymic disorder, two of the six starred symptoms must be present.

Asking about the Symptoms of Depression

The main difficulty for beginning clinicians is in translating the *DSM-IV* terminology into language that is meaningful for the patient. A related difficulty is distinguishing true-positive from false-positive responses to questions about symptoms. Most people experience some of the symptoms of major depression to some degree at some time. Establishing that your patient has symptoms severe enough to meet *DSM-IV* criteria takes creativity, persistence, and experience.

In this chapter, I discuss techniques for assessing each of the NVSs in turn. First, here are some general tips:

- Establish that the symptom is truly a change from baseline. Many patients may have difficulties with concentration, energy, appetite, and so forth, that may be chronic and have little to do with depression. If so, these symptoms cannot "count" toward your diagnosis of a major depressive episode.

CLINICAL VIGNETTE

An intern was interviewing a 45-year-old nightclub owner. When asked, "How have you been sleeping for the past 2 weeks?" the patient responded, "Terribly. I can't fall asleep before 4 a.m., and then I get up at 10. I'm always tired." The resident considered this statement sufficient to meet criteria for the insomnia of depression, until the patient mentioned that this had been his sleep pattern for the past 6 years, and that it had been unchanged over the past 2 weeks. The patient was referred to a sleep clinic and was eventually diagnosed with sleep apnea.

- Establish that the symptom has occurred almost every day for 2 weeks. Many patients may react to upsetting events with a few days of NVSs. This does not constitute a major depressive episode, though it may be an adjustment disorder with depressed mood. It's useful to remind patients that you are asking about a specific period.

  Think back carefully: Have you felt depressed pretty much every day over the past 2 weeks?

- Try not to ask leading questions. An example of a leading question is "Has your depression made it hard for you to concentrate?" This implies that decreased concentration would be expected, and a suggestible or malingering patient might answer with a false "yes." An example of a nonleading question would be "Do you think your concentration has been better or worse than normal over the past 2 weeks?" Of course, you can substitute any of the NVSs for "concentration" in this template.

Screening Questions

> *Are you depressed?*

One study showed that this simple question had 100% sensitivity and specificity in diagnosing major depression in the terminally ill, outperforming elaborate screening instruments such as the Beck Depression Inventory (Chochinov et al. 1997).

> *How has your mood been recently?*

This is a nonleading question, but note that it is more specific than asking, "How have you been doing?" or even, "How have you been feeling?" If your patient starts talking about his distress at this point, go to the NVSs of depression. However, if he says "fine," you should move to the more specific question:

> *Have you ever felt very down or depressed, so depressed that your whole life was affected by it for at least 2 weeks?*

Some patients will be clear and convincing that they have never experienced anything like this, in which case you can skip the whole series of SIGECAPS questions and move on to mania. But if the patient is noncommittal, saying, for example, "I've been pretty depressed, but I don't think quite *that* depressed," you should follow up with more questions.

> *Does your mood vary throughout the day?*

Many patients with depression report diurnal variation, the usual pattern being morning dysphoria with progressive improvement of mood throughout the day (Tolle and Goetze 1987).

SIGECAPS Questions

- Sleep disorder

> *Have you been sleeping normally? (A good initial screening question for a sleep problem.)*

What has your sleep pattern been like lately?

(Depending on the adequacy of your patient's response to this question, you may or may not need to follow up with the following questions.)

What time do you lie down to fall asleep?

What time do you actually fall asleep?

(To diagnose difficulty falling asleep.)

Do you sleep through the night, or do you wake up often during the night?

(To diagnose frequent awakenings.)

What time do you usually wake up in the morning?

Do you generally feel rested when you wake up?

Do you feel more or less depressed when you wake up?

How does your mood change as the day goes on?

(To diagnose early morning awakening and diurnal variation in mood.)

Do you sleep more than usual when you get depressed?

Are you sleeping the way you do when you're depressed?

During a typical 24-hour period, how many hours do you think you sleep?

Have you found yourself taking naps during the day?

(To diagnose the hypersomnia of atypical depression.)

- Interest deficit (anhedonia): Anhedonia is a surprisingly difficult symptom to ascertain. Obviously, no patient is going to come right out and say, "Doctor, I've been really anhedonic lately." You will more likely hear words like, "I'm bored all the time," "I have no motivation," or "I don't care about anything." One problem is that patients may not understand what we mean if we ask, "Can you describe your interest level?" or "Have you been taking pleasure in things?" A patient may only associate pleasure with extraordinary experiences, such as going on vacation, or she may say she has been taking an interest in things when in fact her level of interest has decreased markedly since the onset of depression. Because of these potential pitfalls, it's important to be specific in your questioning.

Before you felt really sad, what sorts of things would you do for fun or for relaxation?

What sorts of hobbies did you have?

Did you read?

Did you play sports or follow the sports teams?

Did you go out to movies?

Did you go out with friends?

This establishes a baseline against which to compare the depressed period. You can then go on to ask about how the depression has affected the patient's activities:

Since you have felt depressed, have you noticed that you've been any less interested in these pursuits?

Have you found that you've been able to enjoy the things that you used to be able to enjoy?

Have you given up doing anything that you normally like to do?

▼ HOT TIP

It is often helpful to ask more specific questions than these three, based on your knowledge of the patient:

Has your sex life suffered at all since you became depressed?

Have you been able to enjoy your pets, grandchildren, or other interests? (Depending on the patient.)

• Guilt, worthlessness, hopelessness: Here, you want to get a sense of how negatively the patient feels about himself. Starting with questions that assess the patient's self-worth often works well:

How have you been feeling about yourself, in terms of self-esteem, since you've been depressed?

Do you feel that you are essentially a good person, or do you have your doubts?

Have you felt especially critical of yourself lately?

These questions touch specifically on the theme of hope-lessness:

How do you see your future?

Do you have hope that things will get better, or does it look pretty bleak?

Do you feel helpless to change your situation?

HOT TIP

In assessing guilt, simply asking, "Do you feel guilty?" may not be enough, because the patient may not be feeling guilty at that moment, even if she's been feeling guilty frequently over the last few weeks. For this reason, it is helpful to ask about some specific aspects of living that depressed people often feel guilty about.

Have you been feeling guilty or regretful about things that you've done or haven't done? Like not being pro-ductive, not reaching your potential, being a burden?

• Energy deficit: Begin with a screening question.

How has your energy level been over the past couple of weeks?

If the patient answers "Lousy," make sure that the low energy coincides with the onset of the depression, rather than being a constant feature of her physical state.

Is this a change for you? Did you feel significantly more energetic before your depression?

Because medical illness can cause anergia in the absence of depression, you may be misled about the source of the loss of energy, particularly when dealing with patients with chronic medical illnesses or geriatric patients. In such cases, asking about the *pattern* of energy throughout the day is helpful. Patients with medical illnesses are at their most energetic when they wake up and then feel worse as the day progresses, whereas depressed patients often wake up feel-ing low and anergic and feel better later in the day.

When is your low point?

When you wake up in the morning, do you feel like you have the energy you need to carry you through your day?

Do you pick up as the day goes on, or do you run out of steam?

- Concentration deficit

   Have you been able to focus on things well?

   How has your concentration been?

   (These general questions are sometimes sufficient for screening purposes.)

   Have you felt more absentminded than usual?

   Have you noticed any changes in your memory?

   (These get at the pseudodementia sometimes seen in depression.)

   Have you had problems making decisions?

   Sometimes, the first sign of concentration problems is a difficulty making basic decisions such as "What should I make for dinner?" or "Should I go out tonight or not?"

   If you were to sit down with a newspaper in front of you, would you be able to read an entire article from start to finish without losing your concentration, or do you have to read the same sentence over and over again?

   Can you watch a half-hour television show from start to finish without losing your focus?

   Have you noticed that you haven't been able to get quite as much done at work as before?

   Concentration questions such as these can be tailored to the patient, depending on what sorts of activities he normally engages in. One study of 31 depressed patients found that the activities most commonly reported to be impaired were television watching (71%), reading (68%), and household jobs (65%) (Pilowsky and Boulton 1970).

- Appetite

 KEY POINT

We are often taught to look mainly for loss of appetite and consequent weight loss in depression, with the exceptions of atypical depression and SAD. However, studies show that weight gain is quite common in typical major depression as well (Stunkard et al. 1990; Weissenburger et al. 1986). In one study of 93 patients with typical depression, 37% gained weight, 32% lost weight, and 31% showed no change in weight (Weissenburger et al. 1986), so you'll want to make sure to phrase your appetite question in a nonleading way.

Since you've been depressed, have you noticed that your appetite has increased, decreased, or stayed about the same?

Have you lost or gained weight since you've been depressed?

Do your clothes fit you differently?

What have you been eating?

How many meals a day do you eat?

These questions often lead to more accurate information; you can quantitate how much the patient is actually eating, and the patient may in fact be surprised to realize that he has been eating less or more than usual.

Does food taste good to you?

Depressed patients sometimes identify their eating problem not so much as a decrease in appetite, but as a sense that food has become tasteless and unenjoyable, "like cardboard," as one patient told me.

Are you eating as if you're depressed?

This is a useful question for patients with recurrent depression who know that their eating always changes when they become depressed.

HOT TIP

This part of the interview provides a natural transition for asking about symptoms of eating disorders. For example, if a patient tells you that she overeats when depressed, ask if she binges and purges as well (see Chapter 25).

- Psychomotor agitation and retardation: Although the *DSM-IV* specifies that psychomotor agitation and retardation should be diagnosed based on what you observe in the patient during the evaluation, the following questions may also be helpful:

> *Sometimes when people get depressed, they notice that their movements really slow down, almost as though their limbs are made of lead. Has that happened to you? (For psychomotor retardation.)*

> *Have you been more restless than usual? Have you been pacing, wringing your hands, unable to sit down for long? (For psychomotor agitation.)*

- Suicidality (see Chapter 20)

OTHER DEPRESSIVE SYNDROMES

Dysthymia

Mnemonic: ACHEWS. Two of these six, with depressed mood, for 2 years are indicative of dysthymia.

Appetite disorder (either decreased or increased appetite)

Concentration deficit

Hopelessness

Energy deficit

Worthlessness

Sleep disorder (either increased or decreased sleep)

The dysthymic patient is "allergic" to happiness; hence, the mnemonic refers to a dysthymic patient's (misspelled) sneezes (achoos), brought on by exposure to happiness. To meet the criteria, the patient must have 2 years of depressed mood, along with two of the six symptoms in the list.

Dysthymia is often diagnosed early in the interview in the context of the chief complaint. When a patient presents with symptoms of depression, a good screening question for dysthymia is

> *When was the last time you remember not feeling depressed?*

The typical dysthymic patient will answer "many years." In fact, the average duration of the disorder is 16 years (Klein et al. 1993).

Along with depressed mood, you also have to establish the continuous presence of at least two of the ACHEW symptoms for 2 years or more. The most efficient way to do this is to start with depressive symptoms that your patient has already mentioned, rather than going through your list. Thus, if you have already heard about her lethargy, ask about that:

> *Over these last 2 years, in which you say you've been depressed, has your energy been low most of the time?*

Atypical Depression

Atypical depression is a depressive subtype characterized by "reverse" NVSs (e.g., *increased* appetite rather than anorexia and *increased* need for sleep rather than insomnia), mood reactivity (the ability to be cheered up by positive events), a pattern of rejection sensitivity throughout one's adult life, and a feeling of being weighed down ("leaden paralysis"). Distinguishing atypical depression from classic depression is important because patients with atypical depression may respond better to monoamine oxidase inhibitor medication than to more typical antidepressants. The patient with atypical depression must have

- Mood reactivity

  When something good happens, does it make you feel better?

  The patient with mood reactivity will answer "Yes."

and two of the following four symptoms:

- Rejection sensitivity

  When someone rejects you, does your mood stay about the same, or do you feel much worse?

- Leaden paralysis

  Does it feel like your arms and legs are heavy, almost like lead?

- Hypersomnia

- Increased appetite

See the section on SIGECAPS, earlier, for questions about these reverse NVSs.

Seasonal Affective Disorder

Once you have established that the patient has episodes of major depression, ask if these episodes follow any seasonal pattern. The most common pattern is depression in the winter and euthymia in the summer.

> *Have you noticed that your depressions consistently come on or get worse in the winter and then go away when the weather improves?*

SAD is similar to atypical depression in that reverse NVSs are usually present, such as carbohydrate craving (with consequent weight gain) and hypersomnia.

If your patient is having a hard time remembering a seasonal aspect to the depression, you can jog his memory by asking

> *Do you generally go on vacation to a sunny place during the winter? Do you find that your mood dramatically improves during the vacation?*

Obviously, anybody's mood improves to some extent during vacation, but the patient with SAD will report a more extreme mood shift that often lasts for several weeks after his return, with a gradual lapsing back into depression thereafter. This mimics the response to light therapy.

Assessing Mood Disorders II: Bipolar Disorder

MANIC EPISODE

DSM-IV Criteria
1. A distinct period of abnormally and persistently elevated, expansive, or irritable mood, lasting at least 1 week, or such a mood of any duration if hospitalization is necessary
2. Persistence of three or more of the following symptoms (four if the mood is only irritable) during the period of mood disturbance:
   Mnemonic: **DIGFAST**
   Distractibility
   Indiscretion (excessive involvement in pleasurable activities that have a high potential for painful)
   Grandiosity or inflated self-esteem
   Flight of ideas or racing thoughts
   Activity increase (increase in goal-directed activity or psychomotor agitation)
   Sleep deficit
   Talkativeness (pressured speech)

Bipolar disorder tends to be underdiagnosed by beginning clinicians. Most patients who present for psychiatric interviews appear demoralized, depressed, or anxious, and one isn't intuitively moved to ask about periods of extreme happiness. It's helpful to realize that bipolar disorder usually presents first as a major depression, and that up to 20% of patients with depression go on to develop bipolar disorder (Blacker and Tsuang 1992).

Even when you *do* remember to ask about mania, there is another roadblock: a high rate of false-positive responses. Many patients report periods of euphoria and high energy that represent normal variations in mood rather than mania. Thus, the most effective screening questions for mania ask about other people's perceptions as well as the patient's self-perception.

In general, you should keep referring to a particular period as you ask your questions, because many people experience the separate diagnostic criteria of mania at various points in their lives (e.g., spending foolishly, talking unusually fast, being unusually distractible), but unless a number of these symptoms have co-occurred during a discrete period (at least 1 week, or 4 days for hypomania), a manic episode cannot be diagnosed.

Screening Questions

> *Have you ever had a period of a week or so in which you felt so happy and energetic that your friends told you that you were talking too fast or that you were behaving differently and strangely?*

If you get a "yes" here, find out when that period was and how long it lasted, and then continually refer to that period when you ask about the diagnostic criteria for mania. If the patient cannot remember such a period lasting an entire week, you should suspect that mania is not the diagnosis. Determine the circumstances of the elevated mood. Being really happy for a couple days after college graduation, for example, is not mania.

> *Has there been a time when you felt just the opposite of depressed, so that for a week or so you felt as if you were on an adrenaline high and could conquer the world?*

The preceding question about mania is handy if you have just finished asking about symptoms of depression.

> *Do you experience wild mood swings in which you feel incredibly good for a week or more and then crash down into a depression?*

Interpret responses to this question cautiously, because some patients who respond with an emphatic "yes" are referring to recurrent episodes of depression without mania or hypomania.

> *Has there been a time when you were so hyper and irritable that you got into arguments with people?*

This gets at the diagnosis of irritable, mixed, or dysphoric mania. Obviously, false-positive responses abound here, and following up with questions establishing that this period of irritability represented a manic episode, rather than a depression or simply a transient foul mood, will be no small task.

> *Has anyone ever called you* manic?

If someone answers "yes" to this, pay close attention. It's not common for normal people to have been called *manic* by someone.

Use DIGFAST to Elicit Diagnostic Criteria

The author of this jewel is unknown, but it's very useful in remembering the diagnostic criteria for a manic episode. The term apparently refers to the speed with which a manic patient would dig a hole if put to the task.

Mnemonic: **DIGFAST**

Distractibility

Indiscretion (*DSM-IV*'s "excessive involvement in pleasurable activities")

Grandiosity

Flight of ideas

Activity increase

Sleep deficit (decreased need for sleep)

Talkativeness (pressured speech)

In addition to expansive mood, the patient must qualify for three of the seven DIGFAST symptoms, or four of seven if the primary mood is irritable.

When you ask about the symptoms of mania, precede your questions with something such as, "During the period last year when you felt high, were you . . .?" This way, you can ensure that all the symptoms have occurred within the same time frame.

HOT TIP

Be sure to ask whether these behaviors occurred in the context of alcohol or drug abuse. If so, you'll have to judge whether the manic behavior is actually secondary to a substance abuse problem or whether the substance abuse is secondary to mania. Unfortunately, this is often a difficult question to sort out.

Distractibility

> *Were you having trouble thinking? Was this because things around you would get you off track?*

KEY POINT

Remember that the distractibility of a manic patient is different from the decreased concentration of a depressed person. A manic is distractible not because his thinking is slowed down, but because his mind is working so quickly and furiously that any mental stimulus, internal or external, knocks him off track.

Indiscretion

> *During the period we've been talking about, how did you spend your time?*

> *Were you doing things that were out of character or unusual for you?*

These are nice questions to start with, because they are relatively unbiased and unlikely to lead the patient to invalid responses.

> *Were you doing things that caused trouble for you or your family?*

This is a good question because it doesn't imply a judgment of the morality of any particular behavior—it merely asks if a behavior has caused trouble for anyone.

> *Were you doing things that showed a lack of judgment, such as driving too quickly, running red lights, or spending too much money?*

> *Did you do anything sexual during this period that was unusual for you?*

KEY POINT

Although you risk pushing a patient's "being judged" button with these questions, most patients respond straightforwardly, especially if the rapport is good. One potential pitfall is assuming that any period of increased spending is diagnostic of a manic episode. In fact, some patients have periods of compulsive buying without mania; such buying may be motivated by a need to reduce feelings of depression or anxiety (Lejoyeux et al. 1997).

Grandiosity

During this period, did you feel especially self-confident, as if you could conquer the world?

Did you have particularly good ideas?

Did you feel that you were right and that everybody else was wrong?

Often, this is a good opportunity to elicit the grandiose delusions that are so common in mania:

Did you feel like you had any special powers?

Did you feel more religious than normal?

Flight of Ideas

Did you have so many ideas that you could barely keep up with them?

Were thoughts racing through your head?

Were other people having a hard time understanding your ideas?

Activity Increase.   The activity increase criterion is similar to indiscretion but focuses specifically on the frenetic nature of the activity.

Were you more active than usual?

Were you constantly starting new projects or hobbies?

Did you have so much energy that you felt it was hard to calm down?

Sleep Deficit

Did you need less sleep than usual?

Did you ever stay up all night doing all kinds of things, such as working on projects or calling people?

 HOT TIP

Be careful not to confuse the sleeplessness of depression or anxiety with mania. Manic patients stay awake because they have so much to think about and do, whereas depressed patients stay awake because they feel tortured by their feelings. Therefore, be sure to ask patients what sorts of things they do when they can't sleep. Manics will report productive activities, whereas depressives will read or watch television as they wait for the solace of sleep.

Talkativeness

Did you find it hard to stop talking?

Did other people tell you that they had trouble understanding you?

Did friends have to interrupt you to get a word in edgewise?

Were you using the phone more than usual?

Other Tips for Diagnosing Mania

- **History of hospitalization:** If a patient was hospitalized during a "hyper" period, chances are good that this was indeed a manic episode.
- **Interview with relatives and friends:** One of the hallmarks of mania is a lack of insight, making verification of historical information particularly important.
- **Family history of bipolar disorder:** Bipolar disorder is one of the most inheritable of all psychiatric disorders (see Chapter 15).

HYPOMANIC EPISODE

DSM-IV **Criteria**

Same as the criteria for manic episode except that

1. The period of expansive or irritable mood need last only 4 days rather than a full week.
2. The episode is not severe enough to cause "marked impairment in social or occupational functioning."

Use the same DIGFAST questions to diagnose hypomania that are used to diagnose mania. The patient with hypomania will describe definite high periods that have not caused real problems in her life. When hypomanic periods alternate with depressed periods, the proper diagnosis is "bipolar II disorder."

Assessing Anxiety Disorders

Screening Questions

- Are you a worrier?
- Have you ever had a panic or anxiety attack?
- Are you uncomfortable in social situations?
- Do you have any special fears, such as fear of insects or of flying?
- Do you have symptoms of obsessive-compulsive disorder, such as needing to wash your hands all the time because you feel dirty, constantly checking things, or having annoying thoughts pop into your head repeatedly?
- Do you have posttraumatic stress disorder, which means having painful memories or dreams of a terrible experience, such as being attacked by someone or surviving a natural disaster?

Recommended time: 3 minutes

Anxiety is a common symptom and can be a frustrating diagnostic issue for beginning interviewers because of the enormous number of disorders that can present with anxiety. For example, many patients with major depression, mania, and schizophrenia also report significant anxiety, even in the absence of a specific anxiety disorder (Boyd 1986).

Nonetheless, it is important to be systematic about diagnosing anxiety disorders, particularly because many disorder-specific psychotherapies have been developed. For example, the cognitive-behavioral approach to the treatment of panic disorder is very different from the cognitive-behavioral approach to social phobia (Barlow 1993).

You should develop a systematic approach to asking about the seven major *DSM-IV* anxiety disorders:

1. Panic disorder
2. Agoraphobia
3. GAD

4. Social phobia
5. Specific phobia
6. OCD
7. PTSD

Even if you ask all the right questions, distinguishing among these anxiety disorders, especially the first four, can be tricky. A useful aid is the *DSM-IV Handbook of Differential Diagnosis* (First et al. 1995), which contains excellent tables to guide you in differentiating one disorder from another.

Following are suggested questions for diagnosing the anxiety disorders, along with brief reminders of the diagnostic criteria for each disorder.

PANIC DISORDER

DSM-IV **Criteria**
1. Recurrent unexpected panic attacks (must have four of 13 symptoms)
   Mnemonic for panic attack: **Heart, Breathlessness, Fear**
      Heart cluster: palpitations, chest pain, nausea
      Breathlessness cluster: shortness of breath, choking sensation, dizziness, paresthesias, hot/cold waves
      Fear cluster: fear of dying, fear of going crazy, sweating, shaking, derealization/depersonalization
2. At least one of the attacks has been followed by 1 month (or more) of at least one of the following three:
      Fear of another attack occurring
      Persistent worry about the implications or consequences of the attack
      A significant change in behavior because of the attacks

The first step in diagnosing panic disorder is establishing that your patient has had panic attacks. Remember, however, that a panic attack does not imply panic disorder. In fact, about 35% of normal people report having had a panic attack within the past year (Norton et al. 1986), whereas only 3% of the population will ever develop full-blown panic disorder (Kessler et al. 1994). Panic attacks are often responses to specific situations that people can successfully avoid (e.g., claustrophobia, specific phobias). Panic may signal a disorder other than panic disorder, such as social phobia or PTSD. Finally, many people experience panic and anxiety that are not quite severe enough to meet criteria for a *DSM-IV* disorder.

The initial screening question for panic is straightforward:

> *Have you ever had a panic or anxiety attack?*

Most people have heard the term *panic attack*. However, a positive response to this question requires verification, because many people define a subpanic level of anxiety as a panic attack. This seems especially true of patients with GAD. Such patients may respond, "I'm always having a panic attack. I'm having one right now." Other patients will ask you what you mean by a panic attack. You need to provide a good definition in lay terms to effectively diagnose panic attack:

> *A panic attack is a sudden rush of fear and nervousness in which your heart pounds, you get short of breath, and you're afraid you're going to lose control or even die. Has that ever happened to you?*

In my experience, this question is highly sensitive and specific for diagnosing true panic attack. Patients who hear this definition and say unequivocally, "Oh no, I've been nervous before, but I've never had anything like that," are unlikely to have ever had a panic attack. For patients who answer "yes," ask them to describe the experience:

> *When did you last have one of these attacks? Can you describe that attack for me? What were you doing when it started? How did it make you feel, and how long did it last?*

The best way to assess the clinical significance of a panic attack is to listen to your patient describe one. You will find out which anxiety symptoms are present and whether the attacks have a specific precipitant.

> *When you have these attacks, do you notice any of the following symptoms: sweating, shaking, tingling in your hands or lips, shortness of breath, choking, your heart pounding, chest pain, nausea, or a feeling that you're about to die or go crazy?*

Although I've listed all these symptoms in one paragraph for convenience, you should ask about them one by one, to give your patient time to think about each. Use the symptom cluster technique (heart, breathlessness, fear) to remember each of the symptoms.

> *When you have a panic attack, does it come out of the blue, or do you pretty much know what's going to cause it?*

Remember that, to meet criteria for panic disorder, the panic attacks have to be unexpected (i.e., out of the blue). Otherwise, panic attacks may signify social phobia, if the trigger is a social situation; PTSD, if the trigger is a flashback; agoraphobia, if the trigger is a hard-to-escape place; or a specific phobia with a variety of possible triggers.

> *Has one of these attacks ever woken you up at night?*

> *Do you remember when you had your first panic attack?*

These two questions will increase the specificity of your exploration. If a patient is awakened at night by panic, it's very likely a true, unexpected panic attack. (Some clinicians would also wonder about a history of sexual abuse.) In addition, people with true panic disorders often distinctly remember their first panic attack.

AGORAPHOBIA

DSM-IV **Criteria**
1. Anxiety about being in places or situations from which escape might be difficult or embarrassing
2. Situations are avoided or are endured with marked distress

Agoraphobia usually develops as a complication of panic disorder (American Psychiatric Association 1994). Usually the patient has a few panic attacks and gradually begins to avoid situations that he associates with those attacks, a process termed *phobic avoidance*. The agoraphobic avoids situations in which a quick escape would be difficult. Typical examples include crowded places (e.g., restaurants, stores, trains, buses) and driving a car, especially in heavy traffic or far from home.

> *Have you started to avoid things because of your panic attacks?*

Ask this question of every patient with panic disorder. Agoraphobia accompanies panic disorder so commonly that the *DSM-III-R* describes no diagnosis of agoraphobia without panic disorder.

> *Do you have problems with crowds? Buses or subways?*
> *Restaurants? Bridges? Driving places?*

Be sure not to confuse agoraphobia, a generalized fear of a variety of situations in which escape might be difficult, with a specific phobia of bridges or buses or with PTSD, in which a specific situation reminiscent of a past trauma may provoke a fear response.

> *Do you get anxious when you leave home?*

At its worst, the agoraphobic's world constricts so much that leaving the home is a terrifying prospect.

GENERALIZED ANXIETY DISORDER

DSM-IV **Criteria**
1. Excessive anxiety and worry, occurring more days than not for at least 6 months, about a number of events or activities
2. Difficulty controlling the worry
3. Anxiety associated with at least three of the following six symptoms:
   Mnemonic: Macbeth Frets Constantly Regarding Illicit Sins
   Muscle tension
   Fatigue
   Concentration difficulty
   Restlessness or feeling on edge
   Irritability
   Sleep disturbance

The patient with GAD is the prototypical worrier, who worries about several things for months on end and is incapable of relaxing.

Begin with this screening question:

> *Are you a worrier?*

Like the screening question for panic disorder, this question is exceedingly unlikely to elicit a "no" answer from a true sufferer of GAD.

> *What do you worry about?*

Common topics of generalized anxiety include the health of relatives (especially children), the quality of a romantic relationship, job or school performance, and the possibility that possessions will break down or be stolen. However, certain topics of worry suggest other diagnoses. For example, excessive worry about performance in social situations may indicate social phobia, worry about having a panic attack suggests panic disorder, and excessive worry about bodily sensations points to somatization disorder. Don't make the mistake of overdiagnosing GAD when the actual diagnosis is something more specific.

On the other hand, some patients experience free-floating anxiety without having a particular focus for their worries. Such patients do not meet criteria for GAD or any other anxiety disorder; diagnostic possibilities to consider include major depression, schizophrenia, or a medication side effect such as akathisia (i.e., a feeling of restlessness caused by antipsychotic medication).

> *Over these past few months of worrying, have you noticed that you've been feeling jittery? Irritable? Do you feel tension in your muscles? Do you tire easily? Do you have insomnia? Do you have problems concentrating?*

The *DSM-IV* requires that GAD patients experience at least three of the preceding six NVSs. Otherwise, too many quite happy and functional worriers would be receiving psychiatric diagnoses.

SOCIAL PHOBIA

DSM-IV Criteria
1. A fear of social performance situations in which the person is exposed to unfamiliar people or to possible scrutiny by others
2. Exposure to the feared situation almost invariably provokes anxiety, which may take the form of a panic attack

The social phobic fears embarrassment and humiliation in a range of different public situations, such as public speaking, meeting someone new, or eating in front of others. All of us fear some of these things to some extent, but the social phobic's fear is unusually intense, to the point of having a panic attack. Social phobics will often give you a clue to their condition by being shy and awkward during the interview, avoiding eye contact, and laughing nervously.

The screening question is

> *Are you uncomfortable in social situations?*

You may need to specify the situations you have in mind:

> *I mean situations such as public speaking, asking questions in front of a class, or being at a party or in a meeting.*

If you get a "yes" to the screening question, ask

> *How uncomfortable do you get? Do you get to the point of having a panic attack?*

> *Is this anxiety so intolerable that you would go out of your way to avoid any social situations?*

SPECIFIC PHOBIA

DSM-IV Criteria
1. Excessive and unreasonable fear of a specific object or situation
2. Exposure to the phobic stimulus causes intense anxiety

A specific phobia is easily diagnosed with the questions

> *Do you have any special fears, such as a fear of insects or a fear of flying?*

> *Have you ever had a panic attack when you've been around this thing that you fear?*

If you get positive responses to these questions, you must further establish that the specific phobia interferes significantly with psychosocial functioning.

OBSESSIVE-COMPULSIVE DISORDER

DSM-IV **Criteria**

Mnemonic: Washing and Straightening Make Clean Houses
  Washing
  Straightening
  Mental rituals (e.g., magical words, numbers)
  Checking
  Hoarding

Must have either obsessions or compulsions:

• Obsessions
    Recurrent intrusive thoughts
    Impulses
    Images that cause anxiety and that the person tries to
      ignore or suppress

• Compulsions
    Repeated behaviors or mental acts that the person feels
      driven to perform in response to an obsession
    Behaviors or acts aimed at preventing or reducing
      distress

OCD is a commonly overlooked diagnosis, because patients rarely volunteer such embarrassing symptoms without being asked. Thus, including OCD questions as part of your routine PROS is particularly important.

Begin with the following high-yield screening question:

> *Do you have symptoms of an obsessive-compulsive disorder, such as needing to wash your hands all the time because you feel dirty, constantly checking things, or having annoying thoughts pop into your head over and over?*

Although this may sound like an excessively long question, so much information is packed into it that if you get a flatly confident "no" in response, you are unlikely to find OCD by digging further. A "yes" requires further probing, because patients will often say that they check or wash, but on detailed questioning they may not meet criteria for OCD.

For example, if a patient says that he checks things, you must establish that he is uncomfortably *driven* to do so:

> *When you check to make sure the door is locked, do you feel like you really have to check it, and that if you didn't you'd feel very uncomfortable?*

You must establish that the checking takes up enough of a person's time to significantly interfere with day-to-day activities:

> *How many times do you check the door usually? Is it just once or twice or do you have to check it ten or 20 times to be satisfied that it's locked?*

Patients may present with a number of different types of obsessions and compulsions. You can often ask about obsessions and compulsions in the same question:

> *Do you wash your hands excessively because of worries about dirt or germs?*

> *Do you feel the need to check things around the house because of a fear that bad things might happen if you don't?*

> *Do you feel the need to save every little scrap of paper because of a fear that you'll need them all sometime?*

For mental rituals, ask

> *Do you often find yourself counting things or naming things for no particular reason?*

To determine the degree of functional impairment caused by the symptoms, you can ask

> *How much time do you usually need to get ready to leave the house in the morning?*

A patient with many cleaning and dressing rituals may take 2 to 3 hours or more to get showered and dressed.

POSTTRAUMATIC STRESS DISORDER

DSM-IV **Criteria**
Mnemonic: Remembers Atrocious Nuclear Attacks
1. The person has experienced a traumatic event that involved actual or threatened death or a threat to the physical integrity of self or others.
2. The traumatic event is persistently **R**eexperienced via memories, dreams, flashbacks, or intense distress when the person is exposed to events that are symbolic of the original event.
3. Stimuli associated with the event are persistently **A**voided, for example, avoiding certain activities or thoughts, amnesia for the event.

> 4. The person experiences Numbing of general responsiveness, as in a sense of detachment from others, a restricted range of affect, diminished interest in various activities, or a sense of foreshortened future.
> 5. Increased Arousal occurs: sleep disturbance, irritability, difficulty concentrating, hypervigilance, exaggerated startle response.
> 6. The disturbance lasts at least 1 month.

Because most people have heard of PTSD, the screening question can include the term, along with a brief definition.

> *Do you have posttraumatic stress disorder, which means having memories or dreams of a terrible experience, like being attacked by someone or surviving a natural disaster?*

Researchers have found that listing examples of traumatic events increases patient recall in PTSD (Solomon and Davidson 1997). If your patient answers "no" to such questions, PTSD is unlikely. A positive response requires that you establish the presence of the *DSM-IV* criteria.

> *What sort of experience was it?*

Asking in this general manner, rather than inquiring directly about the experience, gives your patient permission to answer vaguely, which may be all she can tolerate. Remember that a hallmark of PTSD is the need to avoid the memory of the trauma; allow your patient to do this if she needs to.

Once you have established that a traumatic experience occurred, ask about each of the criteria.

- Reexperience (**Remembers**)

> *Does the experience come back to haunt you from time to time?*

> *Have you had nightmares or flashbacks of this experience?*

If your patient doesn't understand what you mean by *flashbacks*, you can elaborate:

> *Do you find that you're remembering the event and you truly feel like you're back there again?*

- Avoidance (Atrocious)

    Do you find yourself avoiding things that you associate with the memory?

    Inquiring about specific activities or situations related to the actual trauma is better than using this general question. For example, if the trauma was a rape, you might ask

    Do you find yourself avoiding going out with men to avoid remembering what happened?

    If the experience was an automobile accident, you might ask

    Do you avoid driving or even getting into cars because of that experience?

- Numbing (Nuclear): The symptoms of numbing are similar to some of the symptoms of depression, especially anhedonia and decreased energy. You may have asked about them earlier in the interview.

    Since the trauma, has your interest in life gone downhill?

    Your patient may describe a diminished range of activities.

    Have friendships suffered? Has it been harder to have feelings for loved ones?

    Has your sense of the future changed?

    A PTSD patient may respond with "I don't see any future" or "I don't even think about the future."

- Arousal (Attacks): As in numbing, many symptoms of hyperarousal are also typical symptoms of major depression, such as insomnia, difficulty concentrating, and irritability. Hypervigilance and a startle response are more specific to PTSD.

    Since the trauma, have you felt hyper and on edge much of the time?

    Do you startle easily?

Assessing Alcohol Dependence and Drug Abuse

Screening Questions

- Do you enjoy a drink now and then?
- Ask **CAGE** questions
- Do you use any recreational drugs, such as marijuana, LSD, or cocaine?

Recommended time: 2 minutes for screening; 5 to 10 minutes for probing, if screen is positive

---

First you take a drink, then the drink takes a drink, then the drink takes you.

F. Scott Fitzgerald

NOTE

In this chapter, I focus on alcohol dependence; most of the points are applicable to drug abuse as well.

In an initial diagnostic interview, you will probably not have time to do a complete assessment of the history, extent, and consequences of a patient's substance abuse problem. Such an assessment requires a full session in itself. What, then, are your more limited goals? There are three:

1. Determine whether your patient meets *DSM-IV* criteria for alcohol/drug dependence or abuse.
2. Get a sense of the severity of the problem.
3. Determine how the alcohol use interacts with any comorbid psychiatric disorders present.

The most important tip for beginners is to be **nonjudgmental**. This requires some soul-searching because most of us have negative prejudices about substance abusers, and we tend to see them as being morally suspect. Be aware of the extent to which you hold such attitudes, and evaluate whether they are accurate. Try to meet with recovered alcoholics. Their stories are often poignant and will help you to develop a more sympathetic and compassionate attitude. Learn about the disease model of alcoholism (Clark 1981). The more you can view alcoholism as similar to the other psychiatric disorders you treat, the fewer prejudices you will retain.

ASSESSMENT TECHNIQUES

Screening Questions

 HOT TIP

The best quick screen for alcoholism remains the tried-and-true CAGE questionnaire (see below; Ewing 1984), in which a positive response to two or more of the items implies a 95% chance of alcohol abuse or dependence. However, one study (Steinweg 1993) suggests that the way interviewers transition to the CAGE questions profoundly affects the questionnaire's sensitivity. Researchers divided 43 confirmed alcoholics into two groups. In group I, the CAGE was introduced with an open-ended question, such as "Do you have a drink now and then?" In group II, patients were first asked to quantitate their alcohol intake with the question, "How much do you drink?" Sensitivity toward the CAGE questions was dramatically higher in group I (95%) than in group II (32%), demonstrating the importance of beginning the screening in a nonjudgmental way.

CAGE questionnaire:

Cut down: "Have you felt you should cut down on your drinking?"

Annoyed: "Have people annoyed you by getting on your case about your drinking?"

Guilty: "Have you ever felt bad or guilty about your drinking?"

Eye-opener: "Have you ever needed to take a drink first thing in the morning to steady your nerves or get rid of a hangover?"

Begin your screen with the nonthreatening question:

Do you enjoy a drink now and then?

If a patient answers, "I never drink," you should ask, "Why not?" Most people of the American culture have a drink occasionally; people who make a point of *not* drinking are uncommon. They may avoid drinking because they are recovered alcoholics, because they have a family member with a serious drinking problem, or for religious or ethical reasons. Most people will answer with something like, "Oh, I have glass of wine with dinner," or "I have a beer when I barbecue." Jump right into the CAGE questions:

Cut down: Have you ever tried to cut down on your drinking?

A cardinal feature of alcoholism is the loss of control over drinking, and this question gets at that issue. If the patient answers "yes," follow up with

What made you decide to cut down?

The answer to this question will likely move you into an exploration of the adverse consequences of drinking that the patient experienced. (See next section.)

Annoyed: Have you ever been annoyed about friends' or family's criticism of your drinking?

The severe alcoholic will not only have been criticized by loved ones for his drinking, but may have completely alienated most important people in his life.

Guilty: Have you ever felt a little guilty about your drinking?

Again, a positive response is an invitation to further exploration.

Eye-opener: Have you ever felt hungover or shaky in the morning and taken a drink to get rid of that feeling?

This behavior is a good indicator of out-of-control drinking. As your final screening question, ask matter-of-factly:

Do you think that you have a drinking problem?

I have been amazed at how many patients answer "no" to all the CAGE questions and then answer "yes" to this one.

If the patient has answered "no" to the CAGE questions and the drinking problem question, and if there were no clues to a drinking problem (e.g., the odor of alcohol on the breath), the patient has no drinking problem, and you can ask the general question:

> *Do you use any recreational drugs, like marijuana, LSD, or cocaine?*

If the patient gives a negative answer to this question, you can move out of the substance abuse area.

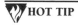 **HOT TIP**

If a patient has admitted to a drinking problem, I have found it useful to ask about other types of substance abuse by using the interviewing technique of symptom expectation:

> *Aside from drinking, what sorts of recreational drugs do you use regularly? Cocaine? Marijuana? Speed? Heroin?*

The phrasing here not only communicates the assumption that your patient has used these drugs, but that he uses them on a regular basis; this is an example of symptom exaggeration. The result is that the patient who abuses these drugs occasionally will feel less ashamed to admit such use (e.g., "I don't use them all the time—I've gone on a few coke binges, and I've shot dope a few times, but I keep it under control").

Probing Questions

DSM-IV Criteria for Alcohol Dependence
The following list refers to the mnemonic: Tempted With Cognac. To be considered alcohol dependent, the patient must meet at least **three** of the following seven criteria:
- Tolerance, that is, a need for increasing amounts of alcohol to achieve intoxication
- Withdrawal syndrome
- Loss of Control of alcohol use (four criteria follow):
    More alcohol ingested than the patient intended
    Unsuccessful attempts to cut down
    Much time spent in activities related to obtaining or recovering from the effects of alcohol

Important social, occupational, or recreational activities given up or reduced because of alcohol use

Alcohol use continued despite the patient's knowledge of significant physical or psychological problems caused by its use

DSM-IV Criteria for Alcohol Abuse

A maladaptive pattern of alcohol use leading to clinically significant impairment or distress, as manifested by at least one of the following:

1. Failure to fulfill major role obligations at work, school, or home
2. Recurrent alcohol use in situations in which it is physically hazardous
3. Recurrent alcohol-related legal problems
4. Continued alcohol use despite persistent problems caused by its use

Once your screening questions have established that your patient has a substance abuse problem, your next step is to use probing questions to definitively establish the *DSM-IV* substance dependence or abuse diagnosis, and to assess severity. One way to approach establishing the diagnosis would be to go down the list of criteria, beginning with tolerance, and to simply ask about each one. While this may be time-efficient, it tends to produce unreliable information, particularly in the patient who is ashamed of her addiction or is trying to hide the extent of it for other reasons.

The better approach is to ask open-ended questions about your patient's drinking history and transition to specific questions about *DSM-IV* criteria as you go along.

> *Do you remember your first drink?*

Alcoholics often remember their first drink vividly, and get a twinkle in their eye. For some, this was the first time they ever felt at peace with themselves.

> *When did you start drinking frequently?*

KEY POINT

The earlier alcoholism began, the more severe and refractory the problem is likely to have become. Recent findings indicate that 25% of male drinkers have an early-onset form of alcoholism called *type II* alcoholism. This is usually inherited from the father, and is a particularly severe form of the disorder, with a high prevalence of violence and comorbid depression and suicidality.

When were you drinking most heavily?

This question allows you to ascertain the sorts of life situations that have been most associated with heavy drinking, and it also serves as a good jumping-off point for a series of questions relating to tolerance, withdrawal, and adverse consequences.

Have you found that you've needed more drinks to get the same high?

Frequent drinkers develop tolerance to the effects of alcohol. A general rule of thumb is that a nonalcoholic person will feel drunk after consuming three to four average drinks on an empty stomach over the course of an hour (Clark 1981). An alcoholic may require two or three times that amount.

When you've cut down or stopped drinking for a few days, have you developed problems such as insomnia, the shakes, or convulsions?

You should become familiar with the usual time course and the symptoms of alcohol withdrawal. Patients generally repeat patterns of withdrawal that they have experienced in the past. This is important for you to know so that you can decide whether to recommend inpatient detoxification to a patient who just stopped drinking.

Have you found over the years that you've had trouble controlling your intake of alcohol?

This is essentially a rephrasing of the "cut down" question of the CAGE, and it gets at the crucial issue of lack of control of alcohol intake, as expressed in criteria 3 and 4 of the *DSM-IV*.

The next few questions are directed toward finding out whether alcohol use has had a negative effect on the patient's life in some *objective* way. I stress *objective* because many alcoholics will deny that they have a *subjective* problem; via skillful interviewing, you can demonstrate that alcohol has caused problems. In this way, your assessment can, in itself, contribute toward the earliest stage of alcoholism treatment, in which the alcoholic accepts that he *has* a problem.

In an insightful and cooperative patient, you can get reliable information about adverse effects by asking straightforward questions:

> *How has your alcoholism affected your relationships? Your work? Other aspects of your life? Have you gotten into fights or been arrested because of your drinking?*

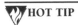 **HOT TIP**

When interviewing a patient in denial, however, you will have to obtain this information indirectly, via the social history and medical history. A severe alcoholic's social history will be replete with failed relationships, job changes, and legal difficulties, and his medical history will be significant for emergency room visits or hospitalizations for alcohol-related injuries. As you glean such information, gingerly introduce the issue of alcohol use:

> *You must have felt pretty down when your wife left you. Was drinking any solace for you then?*

Note that this is a normalizing question, with the implicit message: "Anyone in a similar situation might have reached for the bottle; that's not something to be ashamed of." If your patient admits to drinking, follow up with

> *Was your drinking an issue with your wife? Did she leave you because of it?*

You can use the same technique with other aspects of the social history. When you hear some clue of alcoholism-related adverse consequences, ask if alcohol was involved.

Finally, once you've finished getting the remote alcoholism history, you should ask about recent use. This will help you to determine the need for detoxification hospitalization and the extent to which recent alcohol use may be affecting the patient's mental status. For these questions, you should try to ascertain quantity of both the amount consumed and the frequency.

> *I need to know about how much you've been drinking over the past 2 weeks so that I can come up with some good treatment ideas for you. How many fifths have you been able to put away per day—one? two? more?*

This question combines a number of defusing strategies. First, you introduce the question by saying why you're asking it, not to condemn the patient, but to help him. Second, you appeal to his narcissism by saying "How many fifths have you *been able* to put away?" Finally, you use symptom exaggeration by suggesting a degree of use higher than you expect: one, two, or more fifths per day.

Special Techniques in Dual Diagnosis

If your patient has a substance abuse problem, chances are high that he has another psychiatric disorder, as well. According to the largest American epidemiologic study to look at this question, 37% of alcoholics and 53% of drug abusers have had another psychiatric disorder at some point in their lives (Regier et al. 1990). Using a particularly common example, that of depression combined with alcoholism, two disorders can interact with each other in two ways: Depression can drive a person to drink, or drinking can cause depression, either directly via a depressant effect on the nerve cells or indirectly, via the psychosocial chaos that alcoholism causes.

   Patients with dual diagnoses are complicated, and you may need to schedule two sessions to complete your diagnostic assessment. Here are some suggestions for making these assessments easier. For ease of presentation, I use the example of depression and alcoholism, but any other dual diagnoses can be approached similarly.

   When was your longest period of sobriety?

You want to identify a period of sobriety lasting at least 2 months, preferably longer. Refer to that period in further questions.

   How was your life going during that period? Were you suffering from depression or anxiety?

Try to determine if the patient met *DSM-IV* criteria for a major depressive episode during her sobriety. It doesn't count if she was depressed for only a few weeks after she stopped drinking, and the depression resolved on its own. That's the typical course of alcohol-induced depression. Look for depression that was separated from their alcohol use by at least 1 month.

   Why did you begin drinking again?

> *Was it because of depression, or just because the temptation to drink was too great?*

> *Which do you think is a bigger problem for you, alcohol dependence or depression?*

Sometimes the patient will have a good sense as to which disorder is his central problem. However, you should be wary of the antisocial patient who tries to convince you that he is depressed (rather than alcoholic) to obtain disability benefits or a psychiatric admission.

25 ▼ Assessing Psychotic Disorders

Screening Questions

- Have you had any experiences like dreaming when you're awake?
- Have you had any strange or odd experiences lately that you can't explain?
- Do you ever hear or see things that other people can't hear or see?
- Do ever feel that people are bothering you or trying to harm you?
- Does it seem that strangers look at you a lot or make comments about you?

Recommended time: 2 minutes for screening; 5 to 10 minutes for probing if screen is positive

---

A body seriously out of equilibrium, either with itself or with its environment, perishes outright. Not so a mind. Madness and suffering can set themselves no limit.

George Santayana

The first important point for novice interviewers is that psychosis and schizophrenia are not interchangeable. *Psychosis* is a general term referring to disordered processing of thought and impaired grasp of reality. As such, psychosis can occur as a part of many psychiatric syndromes other than schizophrenia, including

- Depression
- Mania
- Overwhelming stress (*brief reactive psychosis*)
- Dissociative disorders
- Dementia and delirium
- Substance intoxication or withdrawal
- PDs

In terms of the rapid diagnostic evaluation, this means that you must ask every patient you interview, not only those that you suspect of having schizophrenia, screening questions about psychotic ideation.

The second useful point, related to the first, is that there are two types of psychotic patients: (a) those who are obviously psychotic and (b) those whose psychoses are not obvious. In most outpatient settings, the typical patient will not appear psychotic at first glance. He will speak coherently, will not volunteer any delusional material, and will not appear to be hallucinating. However, many of these patients will have a subtle or hidden psychosis that will require a number of screening questions to uncover. These screening questions and techniques are described in the first part of this chapter.

On the other hand, patients who *are* obviously psychotic don't require subtle screening questions. Instead, you will ask probing questions to better understand the precise type of psychosis with which you are dealing. In the second part of this chapter, I define the more common thought disorders and then describe strategies for ascertaining which are present in a particular patient.

GENERAL SCREENING QUESTIONS

When you are interviewing a patient who speaks coherently and has a good grasp of reality, it is tempting to skip questions regarding psychosis. This is a mistake, because hidden psychosis is common, especially in major depression, dementia, and substance abuse. In addition, a nonpsychotic patient may have a history of psychosis, which in turn may influence your diagnosis or treatment.

Two good initial questions are as follows:

> *Have you had any experiences like dreaming when you're awake?*

> *Have you had any strange or odd experiences lately that you can't explain?*

Patients who answer "no" to both of these questions may still be psychotic, and if you suspect this, you should follow up with

> *Do you ever hear or see things that other people can't hear or see?*

This asks directly about auditory and visual hallucinations, but is more graceful than the old standby, "Do you hear voices?"

> *Have people been harassing you or trying to harm you?*

This question screens for paranoid ideation in a nonjudgmental way. You are not asking your patient if she is paranoid, but rather whether she feels others are wronging her. A subtly paranoid patient may welcome this chance to vent her complaints about the FBI's wire-tapping activities.

> *Does it seem that strangers look at you a lot or make comments about you?*

This is a screen for ideas of reference, a common psychotic delusion in which the patient believes that apparently neutral events have a special significance or communication for her. Ideas of reference can be very subtle and difficult to diagnose, as the following vignette illustrates.

CLINICAL VIGNETTE

An intern was admitting a 63-year-old widowed woman with major depression. The patient had become increasingly depressed since her husband died 1 year earlier, and she had not responded to antidepressants thus far, prompting an admission for more intensive diagnostic evaluation and treatment. After establishing criteria for major depression, the intern asked her screening questions for psychotic ideation:

> I: *Do you ever feel that people you don't know are looking at you or making comments about you?*
>
> P: *No.*
>
> I: *Do you ever hear voices or see things that other people can't see?*
>
> P: *No.*
>
> I: *Has anyone been bothering you or harassing you?*
>
> P: *Just the kids in the neighborhood.*
>
> I: *What have they been doing?*
>
> P: *What kids do, yelling and carrying on.*

At this point, the intern was tempted to drop this topic and move on to another section of the interview, but she had a vague sense that there was something more to this story than the "carrying on" of neighborhood kids.

> I: *What sorts of things have the kids been yelling?*

P: *Saying bad things about me.*

I: *What sorts of things?*

P: *Oh, that I'm a prostitute. That I run a whorehouse. They're yelling it day and night.*

As it turned out, the patient had major depression with psychotic features (auditory hallucinations and ideas of reference) and required combination therapy with an antidepressant and a neuroleptic before she improved.

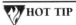 **HOT TIP**

You can also make any of these questions sound less threatening by using smooth transitions and normalization techniques, covered in Chapters 4 and 6.

For example, your patient has just told you how depressed she has been, and you follow up:

> *Deep depression sometimes causes people to have strange experiences, such as hearing voices or feeling that others are trying to harm them. Has that happened to you?*

Of course, you can use many other symptoms as springboards for asking about psychosis, including the following:

- Anxiety: Has your anxiety gotten to the point where your imagination is working in overdrive, so that you hear voices or think people are trying to harm you?
- Substance abuse: Have these drugs ever caused your mind to play tricks on you, such as . . .
- Dementia: When you misplace things around the house, do you ever suspect that someone's been stealing them?

PROBING QUESTIONS:
HOW TO DIAGNOSE SCHIZOPHRENIA

There is both good news and bad news about diagnosing schizophrenia. The good news is that it is fairly easy; the bad news is that we have made it seem complicated by creating a plethora of colorful, though confusing, terms for describing psychosis. To illustrate, here is a partial list of terms in current use:

- Tangentiality
- Circumstantiality
- Distractibility
- Derailment
- Looseness of associations
- Disjointed speech
- Flight of ideas
- Pressure of speech
- Racing thoughts
- Word salad
- Incoherence
- Loss of goal
- Illogical thinking
- Rambling
- Thought blocking
- Poverty of speech
- Poverty of thought
- Poverty of content
- Non sequiturs
- Perseveration
- Clanging
- Neologism
- Paraphasias
- Echolalia
- Stilted speech
- Self-reference
- Persecutory (paranoid) delusions
- Delusion of jealousy
- Erotomania
- Delusion of control
- Delusion of guilt or sin
- Delusion of grandiosity
- Delusion of mind reading
- Ideas of reference
- Delusion of replacement
- Nihilistic delusion
- Somatic delusion
- Thought broadcasting
- Thought insertion
- Thought withdrawal
- Magical thinking

- Poor reality testing
- Attending to internal stimuli

To begin to simplify this semantic onslaught, it's helpful to review the basic criteria for schizophrenia.

SCHIZOPHRENIA

> *DSM-IV* Criteria
> (Requires two symptoms for 1 month, plus 5 months of prodromal or residual symptoms.)
> Mnemonic: Delusions Herald Schizophrenic's Bad News
>> Delusions
>> Hallucinations
>> Speech disorganization
>> Behavior disorganization
>> Negative symptoms

Delusions (Disorders of Thought Content)

A common and useful distinction is made between TC and TP. Both TC and TP can be impaired in psychosis. Impaired TP is covered under the speech disorganization criterion for schizophrenia later in this chapter. *Impaired TC* refers to delusional thinking. A *delusion* is a belief about the world that most people would agree is impossible. Most delusions fit into two broad categories: paranoid delusions and grandiose delusions.

Paranoid Delusions.   According to a World Health Organization study of 811 schizophrenics worldwide (McKenna 1994), paranoia was the most common single delusion, affecting 60% of patients. Paranoid patients believe that people are harassing them, chasing them, spying on them, spreading rumors about them, or trying to kill them. Large organizations are frequently thought to be involved, such as the FBI, CIA, or the Mafia. For example, a young man believed that his wife was an undercover FBI agent determined to kill him for having "blown her cover."

A number of subcategories of paranoid delusions may or may not be present in a particular psychotic patient.

DELUSIONS (OR IDEAS) OF REFERENCE

The patient having delusions of reference believes that casual events have a special (and usually dangerous) significance in reference to her. Thus, strangers waiting at a subway stop may be thought to be staring at or talking about her. In its more severe form, the patient may believe that people on radio or TV are discussing him or speaking directly to him.

NOTE

Delusions of reference can also occur as a feature of grandiose delusions but are most common in paranoia. For example, a woman thought she was being pursued by a hit squad. At work, she noted that coworkers appeared to be whispering things about the plot against her. While she was driving, she perceived an elaborate system of communication among other cars, in which turn signals and headlights were used to indicate her precise location to the killers.

Following are questions for delusions of reference:

> *Have you noticed that strangers on the street have been looking at you or talking about you?*
>
> *Have you felt that people on radio or TV were talking about you in their reports, or giving you special messages?*
>
> *Do you get any messages from books or newspapers?*

DELUSIONS OF CONTROL OR INFLUENCE

The patient with delusions of control believes he is being controlled by some outside force. For example, an immigrant from Latin America believed he was being forced to stay in the United States by the President, who he believed was transmitting ensnaring rays through his television set.

DELUSIONS OF REPLACEMENT (CAPGRAS SYNDROME)

A delusion of replacement is a belief that important people in your life have been replaced by impostors. For example, a woman believed that her mother had been replaced by a stranger who was in league with a fringe religious group attempting to seize possession of her home.

DELUSIONS OF JEALOUSY

A delusion of jealousy is a belief that one's spouse is unfaithful, despite no supporting evidence.

SOMATIC DELUSIONS

The patient having somatic delusions believes that she has an illness or is being poisoned despite the absence of medical evidence. If you suspect somatic delusions, you can elicit them with these questions:

> *Are you worried about your body?*
>
> *Do you think you have cancer or another serious disease?*
>
> *Do you suspect that someone has poisoned you?*
>
> *Has anyone been altering your medication?*
>
> *Is a particular person responsible for your physical symptoms?*

NOTE

Many of these questions are also appropriate for assessing somatization disorder, which is not a psychotic disorder.

Somatic delusions frequently occur as an associated feature of depression.

CLINICAL VIGNETTE

A 38-year-old married woman presented to the emergency room with symptoms of anxiety and depression. In the interview, she said she was afraid that she had HIV infection and syphilis, despite several recent normal blood test results. These fears began after an extramarital affair in which her partner had not used a condom. The patient began to ruminate about the possibility that she had contracted a venereal disease. She became convinced that her entire neighborhood knew about it and that, because of this, she had brought "doom" upon her family. These fears led her to consider overdosing on medication as a suicide attempt.

Grandiose Delusions.   Often seen during a manic episode, grandiose delusions entail the belief that one has special powers and is accomplishing (or will accomplish) extraordinary things. Two common types of grandiosity exist: religious and technological.

RELIGIOUS DELUSIONS

A religious delusion is a very common type of grandiose delusion in which the patient believes she is God-like. In an example of this, a 40-year-old woman was evaluated in the emergency room after having been found standing in the middle of traffic holding her hands high above her head, palms facing oncoming cars. She explained this behavior by saying she was the Messiah and was healing all the people in their cars during rush hour.

The following questions are for religious delusions:

> *Do you consider yourself to be a religious person?*
>
> *Do you have a special relationship with God?*
>
> *Do you have any special religious powers or abilities?*

TECHNOLOGICAL DELUSIONS

The patient with technological delusions believes that he is somehow connected to computers or other electrical appliances, allowing him to exert immense power. For example, a 30-year-old former taxi driver described a business idea. He proposed to coordinate large fleets of taxis that would be in business with restaurants, theaters, and workplaces in a large city. Because all of these settings had financial stakes in people's arriving and leaving, they would be happy to pay the patient for his services. "I wouldn't need any staff," he continued. "I could do it all myself, through the license plates." His intention was to have a transmitter inserted into his brain that could send messages to each cabbie via receivers in the license plates. In an effort to reality test, it was pointed out to him that no such device existed. He responded, "I have it already," pointing to what looked like a large pimple on his forehead.

General Interviewing Tips for Asking about Delusions

NONJUDGMENTAL QUESTIONS

The general strategy in interviewing patients you suspect to be paranoid is to portray yourself as nonjudgmental. If you come across as critical, you are likely to become part of their delusional system.

> *Has anyone treated you badly or annoyed you in any way that was unusual?*
>
> *Has anyone been paying particular attention to you, watching you, or talking about you?*

Both of these questions imply that you want to become the patient's ally, rather than his enemy.

COUNTERPROJECTIVE STATEMENTS

In some cases, your patient may be so paranoid that he clearly distrusts you, incorporating you into his delusional system. A counterprojective statement can work well here. In it, you explicitly acknowledge and sympathize with your patient's projection (Havens 1986; see also Chapter 3).

CLINICAL VIGNETTE

I: *What brought you into the hospital?*

P: *(looking suspicious): You would know, wouldn't you?*

I: *I don't know. That's why I'm asking.*

P: *I was forced here for surveillance. The Secret Service is involved. That's all I'm saying, because I know my rights.*

I: *(using counterprojective statement): And then here I come, looking all official in my coat and tie, saying I'm a psychiatrist . . . you probably think I'm part of the Secret Service too, which would be understandable.*

P: *Can anyone hear us?*

I: *Nope. The door's closed.*

P: *Okay, here's what happened. (Patient opens up significantly.)*

TECHNIQUES FOR REALITY TESTING

Reality testing refers to your efforts to see how strongly your patient believes in his delusion. It helps you to determine the severity of a psychotic disorder and also will help you monitor the patient's response to treatment. Studies of the natural course of delusions have revealed three phases (Sacks 1974):

1. An initial phase in which the patient is totally convinced of the belief
2. An intermediate, "double-awareness" phase in which the patient begins to question the delusion
3. A nondelusional phase

Sensitive questioning will help you determine just which phase your patient is in. Rather than labeling her belief as delusional, frame the delusion in such a way that it is normalized.

▼ HOT TIP

Frame delusions in terms of the patient's *imagination*.

> *Do you think your imagination has been getting the best of you?*

> *Has your imagination been working in overdrive?*

> *Have you been imagining things?*

Blame it on the *mind*:

> *Has your mind been playing tricks on you lately?*

> *Do you think your mind pulled a fast one on you when you thought that?*

Ask about *fantasy*:

> *Do you think you might have been fantasizing any of this?*

Hallucinations

Hallucinations occur in about half of all schizophrenics (Flaum 1995), but they also commonly occur in depression, bipolar disorder, substance abuse disorders, dissociative disorders, and dementia.

> *Have you had any unusual experiences lately, such as hearing voices when there's no one else around?*

Once you've established the presence of auditory hallucinations, ask in more detail about the quality and content of the voices. Adopting an interested and curious attitude often helps break the patient's guard.

> *I've never heard voices before, and I'm curious what it's like for you. Tell me more about these voices. Is there one voice or more than one? Is it male or female? If I were to put a microphone to the voices, what exactly would I hear?*

Ask specifically if the patient is hearing command hallucinations.

> *Are the voices telling you to do anything?*

> *Are they saying bad things about you, or telling you to*
> *hurt yourself or anyone else?*

Another way to ask about hallucinations is to ask in the context of your questions about depression.

> *Sometimes when people get very depressed, their mind*
> *plays tricks on them, and they think they hear things*
> *that others can't hear. Has that happened to you?*

This diminishes the embarrassing nature of a positive response by normalizing the experience (see Chapter 4).

> *Have you heard, seen, smelled, or felt things that other*
> *people couldn't?*

Here, you are asking about all the major types of hallucinations in one fell swoop: auditory, visual, olfactory, and tactile.

Disorganized Speech

What the *DSM-IV* terms *disorganized speech* is also known as *disorder of thought process* or *formal thought disorder*, because there is a disorder of the form, rather than the content, of thought.

To understand how to recognize a disorder of TP, consider your own thinking style. When you think or talk about something, you do so in a linear and logical way; that is, one thought leads naturally to another. In addition, you normally think your thoughts at a comfortable speed, so that when you are speaking, other people can understand you. Patients with a formal thought disorder do not make sense, because their thinking is neither linear nor logical, and there is often a disorder in the speed of their thoughts.

All of the jargon concerning disorganized speech can be fit into one of two clusters: the looseness of association (LOA) cluster and the velocity cluster.

Looseness of Association Cluster. LOA refers to a veering off from the subject at hand. There is a range of severity of LOA, from *circumstantiality* at one end to *word salad* at the other. A patient who exhibits any one of these qualities to a significant degree fulfills the disorganized speech criteria for schizophrenia.

Although a number of terms describe different degrees of LOA, the most useful thing to do clinically is to document that the patient exhibits LOA; describe it as mild, moderate, or severe; and give a brief example (verbatim from the interview) in the write-up. This will allow you to track the patient's response to treatment and will enable other clinicians who read your notes to compare their observations with yours.

CIRCUMSTANTIALITY
The patient with a circumstantial thinking style makes many digressions in her speech and adds extraneous details. These digressions are usually related, however distantly, to the subject matter at hand, and after a while, the speaker will return to that subject matter. You'll recognize a circumstantial style because you will feel impatient and will be forced to interrupt often and redirect to finish the interview within a reasonable period.

Circumstantiality is not necessarily pathologic. Non-patients who are circumstantial are popularly termed *long-winded*. College lecturers and great storytellers are famous for circumstantiality. Within the realm of the *DSM-IV*, demented or anxious patients will often present with circumstantial style.

TANGENTIALITY
Whereas circumstantial speech is basically understandable, though tedious, tangential speech begins to approach incoherence. Digressions are more abrupt and less obviously relevant to the subject at hand. Unlike the circumstantial patient, the tangential patient will never return to the topic of your question, no matter how long you wait. This usually indicates either psychosis or dementia.

Example

I: *Have you ever been hospitalized before?*

P: *I went into the hospital in 1992 and again in 1993. I'm a wanderer, and where people tell me to go, there I will go. Last night I wandered into the room at the end of the hall here and there were some flies buzzing around. I told the nurse about it but she didn't see that as her job, so I swatted them. Do you have any control over the hygienic circumstances here?*

Here, the patient has veered from the subject of her PPH to that of flies in the unit. However, she is basically coherent and with frequent redirection will be able to give meaningful historical information.

Related Term

Rambling: the same as tangentiality, but it is classically reserved for describing demented patients.

LOOSENESS OF ASSOCIATIONS
LOA is a more severe version of tangentiality. The patient makes statements that lead to other statements in a very loose

way, so that the associative leaps are unclear. There are clearly associations going on somewhere in your patient's mind, but you can't make them out.

Example

> I: *What brings you into the clinic today?*
>
> P: *I don't know. I might be thrown out. Benito Mussolini actually came alive out in the waiting room. I figured it out. There was a picture in a book. If it's not my mother, it could have been Hitler. What if that was one of his armed guards. Mussolini was hanging from a tree! Thank you for letting me reason it out. Oh, that's another thing that I wanted to talk to you about . . . being brainwashed. I didn't buy the Beatles tape, I never did.*

The patient is following some pretty disjointed associations in his brain, and it is unlikely that you will be able to obtain a meaningful history. However, the sentences are grammatically correct and internally coherent.

Related Terms

> *Derailment*: equivalent term.
>
> *Disjointed speech*: equivalent term.
>
> *Loss of goal*: refers to speech that doesn't lead to any particular point and that doesn't come close to answering your question; the cause is generally LOA.
>
> *Flight of ideas*: refers to LOA when thoughts are moving rapidly.
>
> *Racing thoughts*: refers to coherent thoughts that are moving rapidly.

WORD SALAD

Word salad is an extreme version of LOA, in which the changes in topic are so extreme and the associations so loose that the resulting speech is completely incoherent. It differs from LOA in that the digressions occur within a particular sentence, between words, in addition to between sentences.

Example

> I: *How did you end up at the hospital?*
>
> P: *It was a section 8 day. I'm not saying there's a utilitarian. I just had no patience with the curfew system.*
>
> I: *Why did you go to the halfway house?*

P: *I'm helpless as a savant idiot. There was a circulation of their publicity. Would you like it?*

I: *What kind of work did you do?*

P: *I worked in computer electricities. It was a nondilated baccalaureate. I mean a nondiluted baccalaureate.*

In this case, individual sentences make no sense. You feel almost as though your patient is speaking a different language.

Related Terms

Incoherence: the direct consequence of word salad.

Non sequiturs: out-of-context words placed into sentences.

Neologisms: spontaneously made up words that often accompany word salad; "nondiluted baccalaureate" is an example.

Clang associations: associations based on the sounds of words.

Velocity Cluster.

In addition to an impaired ability to associate one thought with another, psychotic patients often show an abnormality in the speed or rate of production of their thoughts. This ranges from *mutism* at one end of the continuum to *flight of ideas* at the other.

MUTISM

A patient exhibiting *mutism* simply will not speak. This may mean that he is having few, if any, thoughts, which can occur as a negative symptom of schizophrenia. It can occur in the catatonia of affective disorders. Mutism may also be a response to a delusional system.

Example

A young woman who was admitted to a psychiatric unit remained mute for several days until she began responding to antipsychotic medication. She later related that she had been told by God that her absolute silence was the only thing preventing the collision of matter with antimatter and the consequent annihilation of the world.

POVERTY OF THOUGHT

Your patient has *poverty of thought* if he offers very little spontaneous speech and if his answers to questions are with the minimum number of words required. You have to distinguish this type of psychotic patient from the angry and resistant patient who is admitted involuntarily to a hospital unit or who is under court order to seek therapy. The psychotic patient will often show other negative symptoms of schizophrenia, such as poor hygiene, flat affect, or a history of social isolation.

Example (from Andreasen 1979)

> I: *Were you working at all before you came to the hospital?*
>
> P: *No.*
>
> I: *What kinds of jobs have you had in the past?*
>
> P: *Oh, some janitor jobs, painting.*
>
> I: *What kind of work do you do?*
>
> P: *I don't. I don't do any kind of work. That's silly.*
>
> I: *How far did you go in school?*
>
> P: *I'm still in eleventh grade.*
>
> I: *How old are you?*
>
> P: *Eighteen.*

Related Terms

> *Poverty of speech*: equivalent.
>
> *Lack of spontaneous speech*: equivalent.
>
> *Thought blocking*: Your patient begins to say something, then stops in midthought and forgets what he was going to say.

Interviewing Strategies

You will recognize poverty of thought easily. You will find yourself asking questions far more frequently than usual, because the patient provides no information beyond a minimal response to each question. It is often difficult in these patients to discover whether there are any positive symptoms of schizophrenia, such as delusions or hallucinations. One way to elicit a flow of spontaneous speech is to ask open-ended and provocative questions about general topics:

> *Do you think O. J. Simpson was guilty or innocent?*
>
> *Who was your favorite teacher in high school?*
>
> *What kind of person are you?*
>
> *Do you believe in God?*

POVERTY OF CONTENT

Your patient may produce a copious amount of speech but somehow communicate very little information or discernible meaning. This is usually because the speech is overly abstract.

I: *Why do you think it would be better for you to move out of your mother's house?*

P: *It would be exactly because of the things we were talking about before, and which I was talking to some of the other counselors about. I think we were talking about supervised housing and that would be related to how I might find another place to live, away from my mother, and that would change who I would communicate with. Of course my mother is a person and she would like to communicate with me, and I communicate with her all the time. I think the difference is that it would be a different situation and in a different place. I would have to talk to my case worker about moving. I'm sure my mother wants it, too.*

You find yourself scratching your head. Your question hasn't been answered, but not because the patient has veered away from the topic of moving, as in LOA. His response has remained on topic, but he hasn't said anything meaningful about it.

Related Term
Perseveration: Your patient talks but dwells on a single idea or preoccupation over and over. This can be seen in both OCD and dementia, as well as in psychosis.

RACING THOUGHTS
Racing thoughts refers to the subjective sense of one's thoughts going so fast that they're hard to keep track of, which may or may not be associated with pressured speech. Some patients who are not talkative report having racing thoughts, often occurring with anxiety. Racing thoughts also occur commonly in substance-abusing patients undergoing detoxification. To ascertain the presence of racing thoughts, ask:

Are you having trouble keeping up with your thoughts?

Are your thoughts moving so quickly that you can't keep up with them?

Related Term
Pressured speech: This is very rapid speech that is difficult to interrupt and is often loud and intense. When racing thoughts are converted directly into the speech, the result is pressured speech, and the diagnosis is almost always mania.

Example
I: *How did you come into the hospital?*

P (while pacing back and forth in her room):   I could
remember taking care of business. I felt like I was
here, there, and everywhere. I know I was not sick,
because a sick human cannot remember everything
there is to remember, like that (she snaps her fin-
gers), and I could, and do you know why? Ask the
Master, the Master is everywhere, the Master knows
everything, the Master is God, and that's why I'm
still here. . . .

FLIGHT OF IDEAS

Flight of ideas is a special case of LOA when the incoherent
associations occur very rapidly. As such, it is not necessarily
equivalent to either *pressured speech*, which can refer to quite
coherent but rapid speech, or *racing thoughts*, which can also
be coherent.

Disorder of Behavior (Disorganized Behavior)

Disorganized behavior is diagnosed primarily by observation
during the interview, although obtaining information from
outside sources is often helpful. Observational clues include
poor grooming, body odor, and bizarre clothing combina-
tions. Another clue can be obtained by asking your patient to
complete a simple task. This can be done in the context of the
cognitive examination (see Chapter 19) or simply by asking
your patient for his insurance or appointment card. A typically disorganized patient will pull out a torn, bulging purse
or wallet and will rummage through a seemingly random
array of material before finding anything.

Paucity of Thought, Affect, and Behavior (Negativism)

Symptoms of schizophrenia have been classically divided into
positive symptoms (e.g., delusions, hallucinations) and *negative* symptoms (e.g., flat affect, apathy, asociality, poverty of
speech) (Andreason 1982). The patient with negative symptoms will tend to say very little, speak slowly, show very little
affect, have few spontaneous movements, and be poorly
groomed. His social history will reflect lack of motivation and
inability to persist in school or work activities. Family members may report that he spends most of his time sitting
around, doing very little and that he has few, if any, friends.

26 ▼ Assessing Dementia and Delirium

Screening Questions

- Orientation
    What's your full name?
    Where are we right now?
    What's today's date?
- Short-term memory
    Repeat these three words: ball, chair, purple. Keep them in mind, because I'm going to ask you to repeat them in a couple of minutes.
- Personal and general information
    Name the last three presidents.
    Who was George Washington? Abraham Lincoln? Martin Luther King, Jr.? Shakespeare?
    When was World War II? When was JFK assassinated?
    What's your address and phone number?
    What are your spouse's/children's/siblings'/parents' names and birthdays?
    When and where were you married?

In Chapter 17, I outline a rapid cognitive examination with components based on studies showing them to be effective in identifying patients with cognitive deficits. In this chapter, I'll show you how to tailor your questions to the patient who may have either delirium or dementia. In **delirium**, attention is impaired, and all of the cognitive processes are therefore also impaired. In **dementia**, attention is intact, but the cognitive processes, particularly memory, are impaired.

With this in mind, let's look at the *DSM-IV* criteria for both dementia and delirium and then review interview techniques for making the diagnoses.

DELIRIUM

***DSM-IV* Delirium**

(Note: The *DSM-IV* specifies a number of different types of delirium, but the core diagnostic criteria as listed below do not change.)

- Disturbance of consciousness (i.e., reduced clarity of awareness of the environment) with reduced ability to focus, sustain, or shift attention
- A change in cognition (e.g., memory deficit, disorientation, language disturbance) or the development of a perceptual disturbance that is not better accounted for by a preexisting dementia
- A disturbance developing over a short period (usually hours to days) and fluctuating during the course of the day

Mnemonic: **Medical FRAT**
- **Medical** cause
- **Fluctuating** course
- **Recent** onset
- **Attentional** impairment
- **Thinking** impairment

Impaired Attention

The key to diagnosing delirium is establishing an impairment in your patient's attention, which is what the *DSM-IV* means by "disturbance of consciousness." A delirious patient has difficulty sustaining his attention for a significant period. As in Chapter 19, I discourage reliance on traditional and unproved tests of attention, such as SSST, and instead encourage you to rely on your patient's ability to respond to routine questions.

Most of your interviews with delirious patients will occur in a hospital setting, often when you have been asked to see the patient by the primary care physician. In such settings, there are two types of delirious patients: the loud and the quiet. The loud delirious patient will typically be rambling incoherently and may be struggling against restraints in an effort to leave the hospital bed or to pull out intravenous lines.

The quiet delirious patient, on the other hand, requires some verbal probing to make a diagnosis. It's often helpful to begin by saying nothing, that is, by walking into the room and observing your patient's behavior. A person with normal cognitive abilities will generally look at you and make some kind of greeting, then wait for you to respond. A delirious patient may glance at you briefly and then pay little attention to you. He may be talking softly to himself. He may be looking all around the room, tracking a hallucinated bird or insect.

Hello, Mr. Brown. What brings you into the hospital?

The patient should be able to answer coherently. If the patient answers incoherently, you have to assess the nature of the incoherence. In many mental disorders, the patient's attention is normal, but the TP or TC is disordered in some way.

Of the following three clinical vignettes, for example, only the third describes true delirium.

CLINICAL VIGNETTE 1

A hospitalized psychotic patient gave me this answer:

> *I got tricked into this, but I won't complain, because exactly at this moment there are stereoscopic beams coming into this room from transmitters, and they are focused on my brain cells. Please stay still, because the beams are coming around you now.*

On further questioning, it was apparent that the patient was suffering a fixed, bizarre, paranoid delusion, but his attention was quite intact.

CLINICAL VIGNETTE 2

Another patient responded with the following:

> *This is no hospital, this is my home, because I can see my granddaughter out there. She was just about to bring me in some tea. Oh, I know you. You're that man they sent in to help me.*

The patient had a profound impairment of short-term memory, secondary to Alzheimer's dementia. She could not remember that she was in a hospital, but her attention was intact.

CLINICAL VIGNETTE 3

A truly delirious patient responded:

> Hello! (He looked up at the ceiling.) Something . . . what is that? (He was quickly oblivious to my presence. I asked again why he was in the hospital.) I'm in the hospital for . . . (He looked confused.) There's something here in the hospital, my son said . . . (He looked at me again as if scrutinizing me, then turned away, again seeming to forget about my presence as he looked at the ceiling.)

The patient seemed to understand my words, but he had no ability to maintain his attention to me or to continue a single train of thought. As it turned out, the patient was in delirium tremens after having abruptly stopped his prescribed Xanax three days earlier.

Change in Cognition

Almost all delirious patients will have great difficulty with the three-object recall task, as their attention is too impaired to register the words in the first place. Visual or auditory hallucinations are also extremely common.

Recent Onset and Fluctuating Course

You have to rely on gathering history from sources other than the patient to ascertain that the onset of the cognitive impairment has been relatively recent (days to weeks), excluding the diagnosis of dementia. With regard to fluctuations in attention, the best way for you to determine this is to examine the patient at least twice during the day. If you can't see the patient again, ask other caregivers to report whether she was able to coherently answer simple questions (e.g., "Why are you here?").

DEMENTIA

DSM-IV **Criteria**
(Note: The *DSM-IV* specifies a number of different types of dementia, but the core diagnostic criteria as listed below do not change.)
Mnemonic: **Memory BREW**
- **Memory** impairment (required)
- **B**ehavior disorganization (i.e., apraxia)
- **R**ecognition impairment (i.e., agnosia)
- **E**xecutive functioning impairment
- **W**ord problems (i.e., aphasia)
At least one of the **BREW** criteria is required.

Interviewing Family Members

Interviews with family members and other informants are vitally important in making the diagnosis of dementia. This is because the patient himself will often deny or minimize his memory problem and, at any rate, a demented patient's self-reported history will be unreliable. Therefore, the best way to diagnose dementia is by combining the MSE with interviews of informants. In fact, studies that have compared the two approaches (the MSE vs. informant questionnaires) have found informant interviews to be the more sensitive of the two (Harwood 1997).

When you interview family members, you should begin by asking them to compare the patient's current cognitive abilities with the patient's abilities of 10 years ago. This will put the focus on a gradual decline in functioning, which is what differentiates dementia from delirium.

The general form of your questioning should follow the format of the Informant Questionnaire on Cognitive Decline in the Elderly (IQCODE; Jorm 1991), from which most of the following questions are derived. Ask the following questions:

Compared with 10 years ago, how is this person at

- Remembering things that have happened recently?
- Remembering where things are usually kept?
- Remembering things about family and friends, such as names, occupations, birthdays, or addresses?

- Making decisions on everyday matters?
- Handling financial matters?
- Finding the right word when talking about things?
- Knowing how to do everyday things around the house, such as cooking and cleaning?

Interviewing the Patient

I suggested an approach to assessing memory in Chapter 19, which I won't repeat here. Remember that before you go too far in your examination, do your basic delirium screen (see above). If the patient is delirious, you won't be able to conclude anything about dementia based on the examination; if the patient is awake and attentive, proceed with the rest of the cognitive examination as outlined in Chapter 19.

In addition to demonstrating a memory impairment, the *DSM-IV* requires that you diagnose at least one of the following specific cognitive impairments (remember the **BREW** mnemonic):

- Behavior disorganization (apraxia): *Behavior disorganization* is defined as difficulty accomplishing simple, everyday activities despite an intact nervous system. Think of it as a kind of behavioral confusion. Apraxic patients may have difficulty getting dressed in the morning because they have forgotten how to button clothes or tie shoes. The best way to determine if this has been a problem is by asking family members questions such as

    Does your father have problems getting dressed on his own?

    Does he need any help with shaving or putting on a tie?

    Can he throw a sandwich together easily?

    You can sometimes assess apraxia during the interview by observing your patient do something (e.g., pulling her hospital registration card from her wallet); or you can ask the patient to write down your office phone number, and observe her ability to procure a piece of paper and pen and correctly write down the number.

    The Folstein MMSE includes a standard three-step command for assessing apraxia:

Now I want to see how well you can follow instructions. I'm going to give you a piece of paper. Take it in your right hand, use both hands to fold it in half, then put it on the floor.

- Recognition impairment (agnosia): This refers to the inability to recognize familiar objects or people. Agnosia for objects is hard to distinguish from word-finding problems. If you have identified something that the patient cannot name, you can ask him what the object is used for. If there is no agnosia, he will be able to tell you. (For example, he may not be able to name a pen but will tell you that it's something used for writing.) Agnosia for people is a sign of relatively severe dementia, and it's best to get this information from family members.

- Executive functioning impairment: Here, you are testing a complex ability—the ability to plan and think abstractly. A deficit in executive functioning will often come through during the history. This is especially true if the patient was employed as the dementia began. You will hear about job difficulties, inefficiencies accomplishing tasks that were once easy, and the like. Occasionally, it may be difficult to distinguish this from the personality changes that occur in dementia. New-onset indifference and irritability can play havoc with job performance, especially in service-oriented jobs.

    To test executive functioning, you can use the three-step command (described earlier). However, the classic screening test for this is the *clock-drawing task*, in which you give the patient a sheet of paper with a circle and a dot in the center, and tell her:

    I'd like you to write in all the numbers of a clock and then to draw in the hands to represent 2:30.

    Demented patients may exhibit a number of different errors, such as bunching numbers too closely together, skipping or repeating numbers, or drawing the hands incorrectly. One potential problem with this task is that performance varies by education (Ainslie 1993). Thus, you should give it only to patients with at least some high school education. Otherwise, you may falsely interpret a poor clock as meaning that a patient is cognitively impaired, when in fact he is merely poorly educated.

- Word problems (aphasia): The most common language problem in dementia is a difficulty finding the right word for something. If present, word-finding difficulty will have become apparent over the course of the interview. In mild cases, the right word seems to be on the tip of the patient's tongue:

I: *Who was George Washington?*

P: *Oh, he was that man, the uh . . . top man of the whole thing.*

I: *What do mean by the "top man"?*

P: *The whole country voted for him.*

I: *Do you mean the "president"?*

P: *Right! The president!*

Of course, it may be hard to distinguish word-finding difficulties from memory impairment. A specific screening test for aphasia is to point out common objects in the room and ask your patient to name them (e.g., your pen, your watch, or a chair). However, doing so will only pick up severe cases of aphasia. Interviewing informants is often an excellent way to pick up an early aphasia.

Assessing Eating Disorders, Somatization Disorder, and Attention-Deficit Hyperactivity Disorder

27

Screening Questions

- Eating disorders: Have you ever thought you were overweight?
- Somatization disorder: Have you had a lot of unexplained illnesses?
- ADHD: When you were young, did you have problems with hyperactivity or with paying attention in school?

EATING DISORDERS

DSM-IV Criteria: Anorexia Nervosa
Mnemonic: Weight Fear Bothers Anorexics
- Refusal to maintain body **W**eight above 85% of expected weight
- Intense **F**ear of gaining weight or becoming fat
- Distorted **B**ody image
- For women: **A**menorrhea (the absence of at least three menstrual cycles)

DSM-IV Criteria: Bulimia Nervosa
Mnemonic: Bulimics Over-Consume Pastries
- Recurrent episodes of **B**inge eating (at least twice a week for 3 months) that feel **O**ut of control
- Excessive **C**oncern with body shape and weight
- **P**urging behaviors, such as self-induced vomiting; misuse of laxatives, diuretics, enemas, or other medications; fasting; or excessive exercise

KEY POINT

Eating disorders are relatively easily diagnosed. The problem is that many clinicians don't ask about them, and many sufferers don't volunteer their symptoms, either because they aren't bothered by them, as in anorexia, or because they're too ashamed of them, as in bulimia. Furthermore, clinicians rarely ask men about eating disorders, even though studies have estimated that 10% to 15% of all patients with eating disorders are men, with an especially high prevalence in gay men (Carlat et al. 1997). Therefore, screening questions for eating disorders should always be included in your PROS.

When time is truly of the essence, you can begin with a direct question:

> *Have you ever had an eating disorder, such as anorexia or bulimia?*

However, if you have the sense that your patient may be particularly ashamed of a suspected eating disorder, a too blunt approach might endanger the therapeutic alliance. In these cases, you can approach the issue more indirectly:

> *Have you ever thought you were overweight?*

If the answer is "no," it is unlikely that your patient has an eating disorder. If the reply is "yes," continue.

> *Have you ever dieted?*

Almost everyone, and women in particular, has dieted at some point. You're probing here for a particularly severe diet, perhaps a starvation diet (i.e., fasting) or a diet in which, for example, the patient ate only salad or fruit.

> *Have you ever weighed much less than people thought you should weigh? What was your lowest weight?*

You want to determine whether it is likely that your patient weighs less than 85% of his IBW. Refer to the weight tables in Appendix A for guidelines.

> *Did you think you were overweight at your lowest weight?*

Anorexic patients will report feeling overweight, even obese, at a weight that is far below IBW. Often, the patient will fixate on a particular body part, such as the thighs or the stomach.

> *Were you afraid of gaining weight?*

> *(For women only.) During the time when you were underweight, were you having regular periods?*

To meet a diagnosis of amenorrhea, the patient must have missed at least three consecutive periods. Of course, amenorrhea has many other causes, and you should ensure that the patient was evaluated by a specialist to rule out pregnancy or endocrinologic problems.

For bulimia, ask

> *Have you ever gone on eating binges, when you've eaten an unusually large amount of food within a 2-hour period and felt that you couldn't control your eating?*

⚡ HOT TIP

You have to be somewhat skeptical of a "yes" answer, because what the patient considers a binge may seem like a normal meal to someone else. Ask your patient to describe the contents of a typical binge and decide whether it seems like an unusually large meal.

If she binges, ask if she has ever purged afterward.

> *After you've binged, have you ever gotten rid of the food in some way, such as vomiting or taking laxatives?*

Establish the frequency of the behavior with a symptom exaggeration question:

> *At the most, how often were you bingeing and purging? Once a day? Twice a day? More?*

You have already asked about body image in the anorexia questions.

SOMATIZATION DISORDER

DSM-IV **Criteria**

Mnemonic: Recipe **4 Pain: Convert 2 stomachs** to **1 sex.**

- There is a history of many physical complaints, beginning before the age of 30.
- Each of the following criteria must have been met:
  1. Four pain symptoms (**4 Pain**)
  2. Two gastrointestinal symptoms (**2 Stomachs**)
  3. One sexual symptom (**1 Sex**)
  4. One pseudoneurologic symptom (**Convert**)
- Each symptom cannot be fully explained by a known medical condition, or, if there *is* a demonstrated medical condition, the impairment is in excess of what would be expected.

An excellent screening question for somatization disorder is

Have you had a lot of unexplained illnesses?

If the patient says "no," you can avoid the probing questions. In truth, a patient with somatization disorder will have likely hinted at the problem when you elicited the HPI, much of which will have been devoted to somatic problems. If so, you can bypass this screening question and move on to a checklist of symptoms. Remember to ask when the symptoms began, because the *DSM-IV* specifies that they must start before age 30.

To expedite the process of asking about particular symptoms, begin with the following focusing comment:

> *I'm going to ask you about a number of different physical symptoms. In the interest of time, I'd like to hear mainly whether you've experienced these within the last few weeks, rather than about the long-term history of the problem.*

Without some statement such as this, many patients will launch into a lengthy history of each symptom, complete with information on all the physicians they have seen and the various laboratory tests that have been conducted. You are unlikely to have either the time or the expertise to fully evaluate the adequacy of previous medical workups.

1. Pain symptoms (must have four)

   Please give me a quick run-down of all the pains you've had in the different parts of your body.

2. Gastrointestinal symptoms (must have two, other than pain)

   I want to ask about some stomach symptoms. Have you had nausea? Vomiting? Bloating or gas? Diarrhea? Do you get sick when you eat certain foods?

3. Sexual/reproductive symptoms (must have one, other than pain)

   Finally, have you had any problems with your sexual life, such as lack of desire or inability to have sex for some reason?

   (For women only.) Have you had irregular periods or excessive bleeding with your periods?

4. Pseudoneurologic (conversion) symptoms (must have one)

   Have you been having any neurologic symptoms, such as problems with vision, hearing, or balance? Have you experienced weakness or numbness or had seizures?

ATTENTION-DEFICIT HYPERACTIVITY DISORDER

DSM-IV **Criteria**
Mnemonic: You'll need a **MOAT** around the classroom for the hyperactive child.
- **M**ovement excess (hyperactivity)
- **O**rganization problems (difficulty finishing tasks)
- **A**ttention problems
- **T**alking impulsively

Either 1 or 2 (must have six of nine disorganization/inattention symptoms or six of nine impulsivity/hyperactivity symptoms):

1. Organization/inattention
   Organization problems
   - Can't organize tasks
   - Loses things needed for tasks
   - Has problems finishing tasks

Attention problems
- Poor focus
- Easily distracted
- Doesn't listen
- Forgets easily
- Makes careless mistakes
- Avoids tasks requiring concentration

2. Impulsivity/hyperactivity symptoms
  - Talks too much
  - Blurts out answers
  - Interrupts others
  - Can't play quietly

Movement excess
  - Fidgets and squirms
  - Leaves seat
  - Is restless
  - Is on the go
  - Can't wait for his turn

3. Some symptoms must have been present before age 7.
4. Symptoms occur in two or more settings, such as school (or work) and at home.

ADHD is one of those disorders, such as panic disorder, that involve a long list of criteria, making it impractical to memorize each one. To make matters more confusing, many of the criteria are so similar as to be redundant (e.g., is there really a difference between "often fails to pay close attention" and "often has difficulty sustaining attention"?). Therefore, as was true for panic disorder, the most rational approach is to clump criteria into meaningful clusters by using a mnemonic, in this case **MOAT**.

To meet the criteria, your patient must have six of nine symptoms of inattention/disorganization *or* six of nine symptoms of hyperactivity/impulsivity.

In this section, I focus on ADHD in adults. Diagnosing ADHD in children is more difficult for a variety of reasons, including the unreliability of self-reporting, the necessity of coordinating reports from teachers and family, and a complicated differential diagnosis (Searight et al. 1995). Nonetheless, even in adults, you should try to establish that the problem began in childhood, because the *DSM-IV* requires onset before age 7 years to qualify for adult ADHD.

KEY POINT

As you ask the following questions, remember that many psychiatric disorders other than ADHD can cause problems of impulsivity or concentration, including substance abuse, depression, mania, and anxiety disorders (Biederman 1991).

> *When you were young, did you have problems with hyperactivity or paying attention in school?*

If the response is positive, ask

> *Do you still have those sorts of problems?*

If the answer is negative, it's probably not worth your time to continue with probing questions to verify an old diagnosis of ADHD. If the answer is positive, move on to questions establishing the diagnosis.

Inattentiveness / Disorganization

> *Do you have a hard time paying attention to things?*
>
> *Do you have trouble concentrating?*

Some patients find that they are able to concentrate on engaging tasks, such as watching a football game or reading a tabloid, but not on tasks that are less fun, such as writing a report at work or studying for school.

> *Are you distractible?*

Because many people will not know what this means, you might need to follow up with

> *Do you know what that means? It means that you can't listen to the teacher if the guy next to you is talking or if something's happening outside the window.*
>
> *Do you have a hard time finishing things?*

Some patients may not think of their problem as inattentiveness, but they do find that they get distracted in the middle of a task and don't finish projects. If the patient's parent is present, ask

> *Was he the type of kid who, if you said, "Go to your room and get your shoes," wouldn't come back because*

he got interested in something else and forgot about the shoes?

Talking Impulsively / Hyperactivity

Were you the class clown?

The typical ADHD patient will break into a smile and say, "Oh yeah, let me tell you . . .," and may describe some choice antics. A variation on this question is

When you were in class, was the teacher always having to say to you, "Now, Johnny, you need to stop doing this or that"?

Some patients will say that they are hyperactive when what they mean is overly energetic, as in a manic episode, or anxious. Ask your patient for his definition:

What do you mean when you say that you're hyperactive?

Provide your own definition, if necessary.

By hyperactive, I mean a feeling that you can't sit still, almost as though you had a little motor running inside you all the time that you can't turn off.

Other specific questions to ask include

Do you have a hard time keeping still?

Do you tend to be fidgety?

Although hyperactivity in children is usually quite observable during an initial session, in adolescents and adults it presents more subtly. You may observe constant foot-tapping or rapid hand gestures. The personality style will often be characteristic—outgoing, chatty, and lively—although these are hardly diagnostic of ADHD and are reminiscent of mania.

To ask about impulsive talking, a good question is

Is it easy for you to sit quietly at meetings or in class, or do you tend to blurt things out a lot?

Rating Scales and Family Interviews.   Interviewing a patient's parents will always make an ADHD diagnosis easier. Often, the parent will say, "Oh yes, he was diagnosed with ADHD in school," and will brandish psychological test reports.

The most common rating scale is the Connors Scale, available through school systems and in most institutional child psychiatry departments. If a parent or spouse is present, complete the scale with him during the initial visit. In addition, give the patient a copy to take home to be filled out by a teacher or employer. Remember that you have to establish that your patient's symptoms occur in at least two different settings to make the diagnosis of ADHD.

Assessing Personality Disorders

The *DSM-IV* emphasizes the medical model of psychiatric disorders. Each disorder is presented as though it were a discrete syndrome that a patient "has," in the same way that she might "have" diabetes or asthma. Most clinicians realize that this is a simplistic view, including those clinicians who wrote the *DSM-IV*, which is why they distinguished axis I from axis II pathology. Axis II, the personality disorders, forces us to recognize that each patient has a personality that interacts and often contributes to the formation of a psychiatric syndrome. Treatment focused solely on axis I disorders, therefore, can go only so far, necessitating an effort to diagnose personality traits and disorders in the initial interview.

Although the presence of a personality disorder doesn't make an axis I disorder any less genuine, it signals to the clinician that conventional treatment approaches, such as medication or symptom-focused psychotherapy, may not be sufficient.

Personality disorders are notoriously difficult to diagnose. It is the rare clinician who can confidently conclude after a single interview that a patient has a personality disorder. Thus, this chapter does not assume that you will be able to diagnose a personality disorder quickly, but rather that you will be able to formulate some good hypotheses. Such hypotheses are usually noted on axis II as "rule out _____ personality disorder."

TWO GENERAL APPROACHES

Two useful strategies are useful for assessing personality disorders in the interview. They are not mutually exclusive, and clinicians commonly use both over the course of the evaluation.

Strategy 1: The Ground-Up Technique

In the ground-up technique, you gradually fashion a picture of your patient's personality by working from the ground up—that is, by learning about her life history chronologically, in the context of the social and family history. As outlined in Chapter 14, the formal social history often begins with a general question about family life.

> *Tell me a bit about what growing up was like for you.*

As you ask chronologic questions about your patient's life, especially those aspects of life that involve interpersonal relationships, try to identify any dysfunctional patterns of relating. Recurrent patterns are the hallmark of personality disorders. Memorize one or two probing questions for each personality disorder (see the following examples), and ask them at appropriate times.

A typical example is the patient who relates a pattern of having had few close friendships throughout the early years of his life. Depending on the patient's behavior toward you during the interview (see the section on Behavioral Clues), you may have some hypotheses about which personality disorder is most likely. Perhaps the patient appears anxious and shy during the interview, leading you to suspect avoidant personality disorder. You would then ask a probing question, such as

> *Have you tended to have few friends in your life because you didn't want to have friends, or because you were scared of getting close to someone who might reject you?*

Using the ground-up technique, you will usually be able to arrive at a good hypothesis for a personality disorder or personality traits.

Consider the following example.

CLINICAL VIGNETTE

The interviewer is asking a patient about his work history:

> I: *What sorts of jobs have you had?*
>
> P: *I've had a whole bunch of different jobs. I don't stick with any one job for very long.*
>
> I: *What usually happens with these jobs?*
>
> P: *I usually quit, because the people I work with end up backstabbing me.*

At this point, the interviewer suspects paranoid personality disorder, and asks the probing questions.

> I: *Have you found in your life that people have turned against you for no good reason?*
>
> P: *Yeah, beginning with my parents.*
>
> I: *Do you tend to think of people in general as being disloyal or dishonest?*
>
> P: *Well, I've found that you just can't trust anyone, because they'll always try to do you in if you let down your guard.*

The interviewer, having established two of the four criteria required to make the diagnosis of paranoid personality disorder, will then go on to ask questions regarding other criteria.

Strategy 2: The Symptom-Window Technique

The symptom-window technique entails beginning with your patient's major symptoms and using them as "windows" for exploring possible roots in personality disorders. This is generally done toward the end of the PPH, by which time you will have identified the major symptoms and delineated the syndromal and treatment history. The next step is to ask questions about events that may have occurred each time the symptoms arose. Were these interpersonal events? Were they related to life transitions? In your judgment, do the symptoms seem to be reasonable responses to the events, or do they seem exaggerated?

The nature of the symptoms per se does little to point to a specific personality disorder, but using the symptoms as windows to the personality is often productive. For example, a major depression can be a product of virtually any of the personality disorders, but each patient will arrive at the depression by a different route. Here are some typical examples:

1. Narcissistic personality disorder: The patient finds that nobody meets his high standards, thereby alienating friends and family, leading to a social isolation that can cause depression.
2. Avoidant personality disorder: The patient avoids friendships for fear of rejection, leading to loneliness and depression.
3. Dependent personality disorder: Patient develops a sense of worthlessness and demoralization because of an

inability to make life decisions without relying on someone else.

4. Borderline personality disorder: A chronic sense of inner emptiness may lead to depression, suicidality, and other problems, such as substance abuse, bulimia, and impulse control disorder.

As an example, assume you are interviewing a patient with major depression who recently considered overdosing on some medication after being rejected by her boyfriend. You suspect borderline personality disorder. You can broach the issue with a referred transition:

> *Earlier, we were talking about your depression and some of the suicidal thoughts you had after your boyfriend left you. Have you reacted in this way to rejection at other times in your life?*

After you've gotten the ball rolling by using the referred transition, you can run through the rest of the criteria, jogging your memory with the mnemonic I DESPAIRR. You can introduce these questions with a remark such as

> *I'd like to ask a few more questions about your personality and the ways that you tend to react to certain situations. I'm interested in learning about what sort of person you've been since your teenage years, not only how you've been over the last few weeks.*

This helps to ensure that your patient answers in terms of enduring personality traits rather than recent symptoms.

⊕ KEY POINT

This last point deserves repeating: A personality disorder refers to a *persisting* pattern of dysfunctional relating styles *over many years*, at least since adolescence or young adulthood. Thus, when you ask about criteria for a personality disorder, make clear to your patient that you're interested in the long-term view. Beginners often forget this and may end up falsely diagnosing a personality disorder when the patient actually is suffering an acute axis I disorder. For example, depressed patients commonly appear irritable, needy, and suicidal, features that could easily lead to the diagnosis of borderline personality disorder. Once the depression clears, such patients may magically shed their axis II pathology.

SPECIFIC PERSONALITY DISORDERS: SELF-STATEMENTS, PROBING QUESTIONS, AND BEHAVIORAL CLUES

I have listed below all ten *DSM-IV* personality disorders. For each, there is a patient "self-statement," which is a hypothetical description that a patient with the given disorder would make about himself. The statements are simplistic and stereotypic and are only meant to be used as memory aids, so that you can dependably fix the main features of each personality disorder in your mind. Two suggested probing questions, along with common behavioral clues that might increase your suspicion of a particular disorder, are listed beneath each statement. Finally, a mnemonic is given for each personality disorder, all of which (except the one for borderline personality disorder) were written by Harold Pinkofsky (1997). If you get positive responses to your probing questions, follow up with more questions related to specific diagnostic criteria, using the mnemonics as aids. As an illustration, I have included questions that can be used for each of the criteria for borderline personality disorder.

Borderline

- Self-statement: "I need people desperately, and when people reject me I fall apart completely. I hate them, and I get suicidal."
- Probing questions:

  Have people often disappointed you in your life?

  When something has gone really wrong in your life, such as losing a job or getting rejected, have you often done something to hurt yourself, such as cutting yourself or overdosing?

- Behavioral clues: May alternatively idealize and devalue you over the course of the interview; may be unusually emotionally labile.

  Mnemonic: I DESPAIRR
  Identity disturbance

  Have you generally been pretty clear about what your goals are in life and what sort of person you are, or do you have trouble knowing who _____ is? (Say patient's name.)

Disordered, unstable affect owing to a marked reactivity of mood

→ DISSOCIATED SYMPTOM SEVERE

Are you a moody person?

Chronic feelings of Emptiness

Do you often feel empty inside?

Recurrent Suicidal behavior, gestures, or threats, or self-mutilating behavior

Looking back, when something has gone really wrong in your life, like losing a job or getting rejected, have you often done something to hurt yourself, such as cutting or overdosing?

Transient, stress-related Paranoid ideation or severe dissociative symptoms

When you're under stress, do you feel you lose touch with your environment or with yourself? During those times, do you feel as if people are ganging up on you?

Frantic efforts to avoid real or imagined Abandonment

When someone abandons or rejects you, how do you react?

Impulsivity in at least two areas that is potentially self-damaging

Do you see yourself as an overly impulsive person?

Have you ever done things that can get you into trouble, such as spending all your money, driving like a maniac, using a lot of drugs, having a lot of sex, and so forth?

Inappropriate, intense Rage or difficulty controlling anger

What do you do when you get angry?

Do you hold it inside or let loose with it so that everybody knows how you're feeling?

A pattern of unstable and intense interpersonal Relationships characterized by alternating extremes of idealization and devaluation

Do your relationships tend to be calm and stable or stormy and unstable, with lots of ups and downs?

Cluster A ("Odd")
Paranoid

- Self-statement: "Others are untrustworthy, and they try to take advantage of me."
- Probing questions:

    Have you often found that people in your life have not been trustworthy?

    Have people turned against you for no good reason?

- Behavioral clues: Patient appears guarded and suspicious; patient answers questions reluctantly and with an air of suspicion.

    Mnemonic: **SUSPECT** (four of these seven)

    Spousal infidelity suspected

    Unforgiving (bears grudges)

    Suspicious of others

    Perceives attacks

    Enemy or friend

    Confiding in others feared

    Threats perceived in benign events

Schizoid

- Self-statement: "I prefer to be alone; my world is completely empty."
- Probing questions:

    Are you a people person, or are you someone who prefers to be alone? (Prefers to be alone.)

    Can you name some things that you really enjoy doing? (Takes pleasure in few, if any, activities.)

- Behavioral clues: Patient appears shy and aloof. Patient seems to be preoccupied, in her own world.

    Mnemonic: **DISTANT** (four of these seven)

    Detached (or flattened) affect

    Indifferent to criticism or praise

    Sexual experiences of little interest

    Tasks (activities) performed solitarily

Absence of close friends

Neither desires nor enjoys close relations

Takes pleasure in few activities

Schizotypal

- Self-statement: "I'd like to have friends but it's hard, because people find me pretty strange."
- Probing questions:

    Do you tend to feel pretty uncomfortable around other people?

    Do you sometimes have ideas that other people don't really understand or find unusual?

- Behavioral clues: Patient appears odd in any number of ways—for example, she may be disheveled, wearing strange clothes, or have odd mannerisms. Patient describes strange ideas that border on psychotic.
  Mnemonic: **ME PECULIAR** (five of these ten)

  Magical thinking or odd beliefs

  Experiences unusual perceptions

  Paranoid ideation

  Eccentric behavior or appearance

  Constricted (or inappropriate) affect

  Unusual (odd) thinking and speech

  Lacks close friends

  Ideas of reference

  Anxiety in social situations

  Rule out psychotic disorder and pervasive developmental disorder

Cluster B ("Dramatic")

Borderline
See the earlier Borderline section.

Antisocial

- Self-statement: "I love to take advantage of other people, and I never feel bad about it."

- Probing questions:

  Do you admire a good scam when you see it?

  Have you ever done anything that could have gotten you in trouble with the law?

- Behavioral clues: The patient is excessively cocky and arrogant. The patient always portrays self as innocent and a victim in violent or criminal circumstances.
  Mnemonic: **CORRUPT** (three of these seven)

  Conformity to law lacking

  Obligations ignored

  Reckless disregard for safety of self or others

  Remorse lacking

  Underhanded (deceitful, lies, cons others)

  Planning insufficient (impulsive)

  Temper

Histrionic

- Self-statement: "I'm quite an emotional and sexually charming person, and I need to be the center of attention!"
- Probing questions:

  Do you like to be the center of attention? (Yes.)

  When you feel an emotion, do you keep it inside or do you express it? (Express it.)

- Behavioral clues: The patient is flamboyantly and seductively groomed or dressed. The patient is rapidly and dramatically self-revealing to the point of inappropriateness, even in the context of a psychiatric evaluation.
  Mnemonic: **PRAISE ME** (five of these eight)

  Provocative (or sexually seductive) behavior

  Relationships (considered more intimate than they are)

  Attention (uncomfortable when not the center of attention)

  Influenced easily

  Style of speech (impressionistic, lacks detail)

  Emotions (rapidly shifting and shallow)

Made up (physical appearance used to draw attention to self)

Emotions exaggerated (theatrical)

Narcissistic

- Self-statement: "I'm an extremely talented and special person, better than most people, and yet I get angry and depressed because people don't recognize how great I am!"
- Probing questions:

    Do you often find yourself getting frustrated because other people don't meet your standards? (Yes.)

    What are your ambitions for yourself? (Will be unrealistically high.)

- Behavioral clues: The patient may appear haughty and excessively critical of your credentials or experience. She may begin the interview with a litany of angry complaints about how unfairly others have treated her.
    Mnemonic: **SPEEECIAL** (five of these nine)

    Special (believes he is special and unique)

    Preoccupied with fantasies (e.g., of unlimited success, power)

    Envious

    Entitlement

    Excessive admiration required

    Conceited

    Interpersonal exploitation

    Arrogant

    Lacks empathy

Cluster C ("Anxious")

Avoidant

- Self-statement: "I'm really afraid of what people will think of me, so I avoid making new friends to prevent rejection."
- Probing questions:

    Do you tend to avoid meeting people or getting close to people? (Yes.)

> *Is that because you prefer to be alone or because you've been rejected before and you don't want it to happen again? (The latter.)*

- Behavioral clues: The patient may appear shy and nervous but with a poignant eagerness to make contact. He may begin the interview reluctant to open up and will typically become quite self-revealing once rapport has been established.
  Mnemonic: **CRINGES** (four of these seven)

  Certainty of being liked required before willing to risk involvement

  Rejection possibility preoccupies his thoughts

  Intimate relationships avoided

  New relationships avoided

  Gets around occupational activities that involve interpersonal contact

  Embarrassment potential prevents new activities

  Self viewed as unappealing, inept, inferior

Dependent

- Self-statement: "I'm pretty passive and dependent on others for direction, and I go far out of my way not to displease people who are important to me."
- Probing questions:

  Do you consider yourself a completely independent person, or have you tended to lean on others in your life for emotional support and guidance? (Lean on someone else.)

  Who has made most major decisions in your life, you or your _____ (spouse, parents, or other, depending on situation)? (Someone other than the patient.)

- Behavioral clues: The patient will seem to make extraordinary attempts to immediately gain your affection.
  Mnemonic: **RELIANCE** (five of these eight)

  Reassurance required for decisions

  Expressing disagreement difficult (because of fear of loss of support or approval)

Life responsibilities assumed by others

Initiating projects difficult

Alone (feels helpless and a sense of discomfort when alone)

Nurturance (goes to excessive lengths to obtain nurturance and support)

Companionship sought urgently when close relationship ends

Exaggerated fears of being left to care for self

Obsessive-Compulsive

- Self-statement: "I'm a perfectionist. I keep lists, I drive myself hard, and I'm very serious about life."
- Probing questions:

    Do you consider yourself a perfectionist?

    Do you drive yourself so hard with your work that you find you have no time for leisure activities?

- Behavioral clues: The patient is meticulously groomed and dressed. He will tend to give an excessively detailed and accurate account of his symptoms.
  Mnemonic: **LAW FIRMS** (four of these eight)

Loses point of activity

Ability to complete tasks compromised by perfectionism

Worthless objects (unable to discard)

Friendships (and leisure activities) excluded (owing to pre-occupation with work)

Inflexible, scrupulous, overconscientious

Reluctant to delegate

Miserly

Stubborn

INTERVIEWING FOR TREATMENT

There came a time when the risk to remain tight in the bud was more painful than the risk it took to blossom.

Anaïs Nin

How to Educate Your Patient

Does this mean I'm crazy?

Is this medication going to turn me into a zombie?

Am I going to be this way for the rest of my life?

These are the sorts of questions that patients will ask you, often toward the end of the diagnostic interview. Clinicians eventually develop an effective approach to answering such questions in lay terms. Although patient education is rarely formally taught in training programs, from the patient's perspective, it is often the most important part of the initial evaluation.

Educating your patient about his disorder is helpful for various reasons. First, education decreases his anxiety. As clinicians, we tend to take mental illness for granted, but patients are often terrified by their disorders. By giving an illness a name and showing that its prognosis and treatment are well understood and that millions of other people have experienced it, we can significantly decrease the patient's anxiety.

Second, patient education improves adherence to treatment, both for medications and therapy. Misconceptions about psychiatric treatment abound in our society; most people get their information about psychiatry from cartoons, television sitcoms, and news magazines, which leads to a mismatch between reality and fantasy. For example, many patients believe that psychotherapy is a long-term process in which painful family dynamics are rehashed for years on end. Such a misconception decreases the likelihood that patients will commit to therapy. When educated about the fact that most present-day therapy is brief and focuses on current problems, patients become more receptive to referrals.

Misinformation about medications also abounds. Patients often believe that antidepressants are to be discontinued once they feel better, as opposed to the 6 to 12 months of continuous therapy recommended. Other patients consider antidepressants to be rapid mood boosters. One patient for whom I had prescribed Prozac for depression came back in a month reporting that she had only "needed to take" the Prozac four or five times. Her belief had been that the medication was to be taken only on those mornings that she awoke feeling very depressed.

In this chapter, I guide you through a commonly used strategy for providing patient education that can be applied to a wide variety of mental disorders.

BRIEFLY STATE YOUR DIAGNOSIS

Although this is self-explanatory, I would add that you needn't always phrase the diagnosis in *DSM-IV* terminology. For example, I often tell patients that they have a "clinical depression" rather than a "major depression," because I know from experience that more patients have heard of the former than the latter.

WHAT YOUR PATIENT KNOWS ABOUT THE DISORDER

The way I generally find out what my patient knows about the disorder is as an extension of providing a diagnosis. Thus:

> *I think that you've been suffering from a clinical, or major, depression. Do you know what that is?*

If the patient says "yes," I ask him to elaborate a bit:

> *What is your definition of depression?*

As a prelude to treatment negotiation, I often ask whether the patient has any expectations about treatment.

> *Do you have any ideas about treatment?*

Some patients may overtly request a particular form of treatment, such as psychotherapy or medication, whereas others may tell you what they *don't* want.

MINI-LECTURE ABOUT THE DISORDER

Not all patients want to hear you wax poetic about their disorders. For example, a well-informed patient who has just delineated each of the *DSM-IV* criteria of OCD might be insulted to hear you repeat them. Other patients may be quite uninformed but, taking the attitude that you, and not they, are the doctor, might feel uncomfortable with your efforts to educate them and involve them in their treatment. There's no firm rule about which patients should get a mini-lecture. Accordingly, you can ask the patient something like this:

> *Would you like me to give you some information on depression?*

Although it is the rare patient who responds with a flat "no," even if he'd prefer not to have the information, you can generally gauge the degree of interest based on the response and adjust the length of your mini-lecture accordingly.

As a guide for structuring your mini-lecture, I turn to the experience of the researchers at the University of Pittsburgh, who used a psychoeducational program that helped them achieve a remarkably high (90%) adherence to treatment over 3 years (Frank et al. 1995; Jacobs et al. 1987). Their program was devised to teach patients and their families about depression. Its components included the following:

- Define the illness. Ask your patient to identify all the symptoms that he has experienced. A chalkboard, or more realistically, a piece of paper on which to write, is helpful. Define the disorder as an illness that has many symptoms, including the ones your patient has identified; try to portray it as an illness similar to the medical illnesses of diabetes or hypertension. This helps decrease the stigma associated with mental illness.
- Discuss the prevalence and course of the illness. (Refer to Appendix A for a pocket card listing the prevalence for the major mental disorders.)
- Discuss the causes. Although we don't know the causes of most mental illnesses, you can discuss some different theories.
- Discuss the options for treatment.
- For medications, discuss side effect profiles and emphasize the fact that individuals experience different side effects.

Here is an example of a mini-lecture for major depression:

A major depression is a breakdown in a person's ability to cope with stress. While we all get sad from time to time when things go poorly, a person with major depression feels so down that the basic functions of living are affected. As with medical illnesses, depression causes specific symptoms. In your case, you haven't been able to sleep, you've lost your appetite, you haven't been able to concentrate at work, and you've had some scary suicidal thoughts.

Depression is quite common; about 10% of people develop it at some point in their lives. What causes it isn't clear. For some people, stressors seem to cause depression; this may be the case for you, since you felt bad after your divorce. In other cases, depression seems to be a biological disorder.

The good news about depression is that it's very treatable. There are two main techniques, medication or talk therapy. A combination of the two is often most effective. In your case, I'd recommend the combined treatment. Do you have any questions about all this?

I'll also give you an example of a mini-lecture for borderline personality disorders, just to prove that you can discuss personality disorders with patients without sounding critical.

I: *You're suffering from borderline personality disorder. Do you know what that is?*

P: *No, but it sounds bad, like being on the edge.*

I: *You're not far off. It is a bit like being on the edge. People with borderline personality disorder tend to have poor self-esteem, and this causes them to be very moody, especially when it comes to dealing with friends and family. For instance, you told me earlier that when people reject you, you don't just get depressed, you get suicidal. And when you get angry at people, you really lose control.*

P: *That's just the way I've always been; I didn't know it was an official disorder.*

I: *It is, and believe me, you're not alone. Studies show that about 2% of all people have the same problem. No one knows exactly what causes it, but the early family environment usually plays a role. The best treatment is long-term therapy, with medications from time to time to treat depression.*

You'll develop your own style of educating patients, and your lecture will inevitably vary depending on the patient. As much as possible, you want to speak your patient's language, which will vary with level of intelligence and education, cultural background, age, and other factors.

QUESTIONS

Even if you are feeling the pressure of the end of the hour, give your patient plenty of time to think about questions.

WRITTEN EDUCATIONAL MATERIALS

Giving written educational materials to your patients allows them to consider the information in privacy and at greater length. You may use the handouts in Appendix B, all of which are public domain documents that can be reproduced with or without acknowledgments.

Negotiating a Treatment Plan

Essential Concepts

- Elicit the patient's agenda.
- Negotiate a plan that you and your patient can agree on.
- Help the patient implement the agreed-on plan.

Once you've come up with a diagnosis, you have to determine a treatment plan based on that diagnosis. A treatment plan is something you should arrive at with your patient, rather than handing it to her like a prescription. The more you involve your patient in planning treatment, the more likely that she will follow through with the plan.

Compliance was once a popular term for describing good follow-up, but now that term is being gradually replaced with *adherence*, which implies less passivity. A patient *chooses* to adhere, while he *is made* to comply. Researchers have found that when clinicians and patients negotiate a treatment plan together, both adherence and clinical outcome are improved (Eisenthal et al. 1979). Lazare et al. (1975) have outlined an approach to negotiating a treatment plan that makes good sense, from which the following schema is adapted.

ELICIT THE PATIENT'S AGENDA

Your patient's agenda may not be as obvious as it first appears. You can begin to elicit it with a simple question, such as

> *How do you hope I can help you?*

Note that this is a less confrontational way of asking about your patient's agenda than asking

> *What do you want?*

> *What do you expect?*

At this point, the patient may answer vaguely or put the ball back in your court:

I want to feel better.

I don't know. You're the doctor.

It's often important to clarify what sort of information you're seeking:

How were you hoping that I could help you to feel better?

 HOT TIP

Often, patients come into an interview with a few specific requests, such as a desire for medication, therapy, a community referral, a letter to their employer, and so on. Some patients may feel embarrassed about divulging their requests so blatantly and may need some encouragement from you:

> *Sometimes patients have a pretty clear idea of what they'd like, for instance medication, counseling, or a piece of advice about something, a letter to someone. (A normalizing response.)*

However, many patients who come to see a clinician really don't have a specific request or agenda. This is often the case with patients who are new to the mental health care system or who are less familiar with the modern consumer model of health care. Don't force the issue with these patients; if they say that they want to hear what your recommendation is and they'll follow it just because you are the expert, go along with it.

NEGOTIATE A PLAN

Remember that eventual treatment adherence is enhanced when the patient and practitioner agree on the nature of the problem. The next phase of negotiation involves arriving at this agreement. If you and your patient agree at the outset about a plan, go directly to the implementation phase. However, often enough you'll find that your patient's request is either unrealistic or not clinically indicated. Thank your stars that you elicited the request with time to spare, because now you must negotiate a mutually agreed-on goal. Each negotiation will be different, depending on the nature of the request. Creativity is a plus.

Common problematic requests, along with possible negotiation strategies, are as follows:

Request: Your patient asks you for medication, but you cannot prescribe.

Strategy: Determine how urgent the need for medication is. If it's not urgent, make a referral to a psychiatrist, and teach the patient a psychological method for symptom relief, such as relaxation exercises, hypnosis, or cognitive restructuring. Now is a good time to reach into your file of patient handouts. If the need is urgent, refer the patient to an emergency room or crisis clinic, leaving enough time for you to call the clinic to inform the psychiatrist of the patient's diagnosis and medication needs.

Request: Your patient asks for inappropriate medication, such as benzodiazepines for someone with a history of benzodiazepine abuse or antidepressants for mild or transient depressive symptoms.

Strategy: Present a mini-lecture about the patient's disorder, complete with handouts and recommendations of books.

Request: The patient seeks hospitalization for a problem that can be treated in an outpatient setting.

Strategy: This has become an increasingly problematic request in our era of managed care, and patients may need some education about this issue:

> *These days, insurance companies rarely pay for hospitalizations unless the patient is suicidal, because we have a lot of outpatient treatments that work well.*

An important thing to keep in mind is the possibility that the patient is suffering much more than she originally indicated, and that her request for hospitalization is her way of obliquely disclosing that. You may need to reassess her for SI at this point. If you're still satisfied that hospitalization is not indicated, discuss some other options, such as

Day hospitalization

Respite care

Staying with a friend or relative for a while if the home situation is intolerable

Taking a few days off from work

Having the patient call you (or another clinician) for daily check-ins during a crisis period

Setting up more frequent appointments

A short course of an antianxiety medication

IMPLEMENTING THE AGREED-ON PLAN

Your agreed-on plan will likely fall into one or both of the following categories:

- A follow-up therapy appointment with you or someone else
- Medication trial

Follow-Up Appointments

Your job is to increase the chances that your patient will show up at the follow-up appointment, regardless of where that is. You've already contributed to this cause by involving the patient in the process of deciding on a plan. What more can you do?

The research shows that the highest follow-up adherence rates occurred under the following circumstances (Eisenthal 1979):

- The wait for follow-up appointments is short.
- Referrals are made to specific clinicians rather than to a clinic.
- Specific appointments are made at the time of disposition.
- The patient speaks directly to someone at the referral clinic during the evaluation session.

The closer you can come to implementing these guidelines, the better. Of course, this requires plenty of preinterview preparation (see Chapter 2 on logistical preparation), including the following:

- Have an efficient system for booking your follow-up appointments.
- Have a list of specific clinicians who do not have excessive waiting periods for appointments.
- Have a list of referral clinics with their phone numbers so your patient can call and make the appointment from your office.

Medication Trials

If you have truly collaborated with your patient in deciding on a medication trial, you're well on your way toward achieving adherence to the regimen. Here are some practical issues regarding medications and suggestions for dealing with them:

1. Determine how your patient will pay for medication. Some insurance companies pay for prescriptions and others don't. If the patient has to pay out of pocket, make sure she knows how much she's going to be spending. As a general guideline, medications that have been released within the last 10 years or so tend to be very expensive. This is particularly true of the new antidepressants, such as the selective serotonin-reuptake inhibitors, which typically cost upwards of $100 per month. If she can't afford that, you may be able to provide your patient with samples, depending on their availability at your clinic. Many drug companies now have voucher programs. Under these programs, the drug company will send you a stack of vouchers, each of which is good for one month's medication. The patient gives the voucher to the pharmacist and gets the medication.

2. Make sure your patient understands the side effect profile of the medication.

3. Simplification increases recall and compliance. Thus, instead of "Take 20 mg of Prozac once a day and 50 mg of trazodone at night, as needed for insomnia," say, "Take the green capsule every morning and the white pill at night if you can't sleep."

4. Having your patient repeat what you say increases her recall of your instructions.

Writing Up the Results of the Interview

I've had a long and stormy relationship with the dreaded write-up. During medical school, the requirement of a novel-length write-up was a welcome reprieve from the stresses of rounding on patients and making oral presentations. In residency, I became annoyed with the write-up, which seemed a pesky intrusion into the limited time I had to spend with patients. At the end of a long day, I would sit down heavily at the Dictaphone and try to gather my thoughts, hoping that the resulting transcription would be coherent.

It wasn't until I had been in clinical practice for a few years that I came to terms with the write-up. Having come full circle, I'm back to (sort of) liking it, viewing it as a welcome few minutes of quiet thought and synthesis between patient appointments.

I hope this chapter will help you to work through some of the more painful moments in your own relationship with the write-up. I outline some formats for you to choose among, and I provide some tips that will help you streamline the process.

Every write-up represents a balancing act among three objectives:

1. Thoroughness
2. Time-efficiency
3. Readability

The ideal write-up will incorporate all three objectives. It will be thorough enough to document the basis for a diagnosis and treatment plan; it will not require so much time that it would be unfeasible for a busy clinician to produce; and it will not be so lengthy as to provoke sighs from equally busy colleagues who must read the write-up because of their involvement in the patient's treatment.

In general, a write-up should not take you more than 10 to 15 minutes to produce, whether you dictate it or write it yourself. It should not be longer than two or three typed pages if you really want colleagues to read it.

IDENTIFYING DATA

The identifying data should be a fairly long initial sentence that sets the stage for the entire evaluation. You want to not only identify who the patient is, but also to locate her within the context of social and cultural norms. This includes age, sex, marital status, and source of referral at a minimum, and may include other information such as occupation, living situation, and presence of other family.

> This is a 45-year-old, twice-married woman with two grown children, who is an accountant for her husband's carpet cleaning business, and who was referred by her primary care doctor because of increasing anxiety and the possibility that she is abusing anxiety and pain medication.

or

> This is a 29-year-old, single, white man on psychiatric disability, living in a group home downtown, with a long history of paranoid schizophrenia, who was admitted to the hospital after group home staff members found him in the process of drinking a bottle of methyl alcohol in an apparent suicide attempt.

CHIEF COMPLAINT

The chief complaint should be a verbatim sentence of the patient's, usually in response to your question as to the reason he is seeking help.

> *My wife made me come here. There's nothing wrong with me.*
>
> *My mother just died. I can't deal with it.*
>
> *I just figured it was time to see a therapist to work out some issues.*

Each of these statements reflects a different sense of purpose and urgency for treatment, and consequently, this information is helpful in setting the stage for the report to follow.

HISTORY OF PRESENT ILLNESS

In Chapter 12, I describe two different definitions of the HPI, one referring to the history of the illness, which may begin years before the interview (history of syndrome approach), and the other referring more narrowly to events of the past few weeks (history of present crisis approach). Which definition to use is a matter of personal or institutional preference. Following are examples of both approaches.

History of Syndrome

Mr. M has a long history of bipolar disorder, beginning in his junior year of college. He was hospitalized for manic behavior, which included studying for days at a time to the point of exhaustion. In addition, he exhibited grandiose, disorganized behavior when he "occupied" the chancellor's outer office, and stated that he was the chancellor of the university. He was started on lithium at that point and did well for several years, until he had a series of hospitalizations in the early 1990s for depression and alcohol use after a divorce from his wife.

His last hospitalization was 2 years ago for depression, and he has done fairly well since then, taking medications (Effexor and Depakote) and going to regular therapy and medication appointments.

History of Present Crisis

Mr. M has a long history of bipolar disorder with several hospitalizations, but had been doing fairly well for the past 2 years until about 2 weeks ago, when his girlfriend noticed a pattern of manic behavior, which began after a promotion to a new position at his company. He has slept an average of 3 hours a night because of a need to "prepare for his day," he has been talking more rapidly than usual, and he has been making unrealistic plans to become the president of his company. He consented to this admission on the advice of his girlfriend and his outpatient caregivers.

PAST PSYCHIATRIC HISTORY

The nature of the PPH section of your write-up depends on how thorough you have been in the HPI. Generally, the PPH is a time to go into some detail on what sort of psychiatric treatment your patient has had in the past. In Chapter 13, I recommend the mnemonic Go CHaMP as a way of organizing your questioning, and you can also use this for your write-up. You can begin with a General statement, such as

> The patient feels that he has received fairly intense, and overall successful, treatment for his depression over the years.

or

> The patient has started treatment at various times but by his own admission has been generally noncompliant.

In CHaMP, the C is for current Caregivers, if any. Documenting Hospitalizations is straightforward, and usually the detail is limited by your patient's memory. Noting the date of the last hospitalization is important, because it has implications for the severity of the current problem. Having a separate heading for "Medication trials" is often very helpful, both for other caregivers and for easy reference if you have to make a medication change several months or years after the first visit. Finally, documentation about past Psychotherapy should include a note about whether the patient found it helpful and why or why not.

SUBSTANCE USE HISTORY

Where in the evaluation should you document history of substance use? This varies by practitioner, with some including it in the PPH, others in the social history, and still others in the medical history, usually under "habits." My preference is to use a main heading devoted to the issue, because it is such an important and often overlooked part of the psychiatric history.

Under substance use, I include tobacco and caffeine use, as well as the usual array of more insidious substances, such as alcohol or cocaine.

REVIEW OF SYMPTOMS

The review of symptoms is where you can really impress your readers with your diagnostic thoroughness. Simply go through the major diagnostic categories, indicating whether the patient met any of the criteria, and excluding those that you already mentioned in the HPI and in the substance abuse section, if you have included one.

> On review of psychiatric symptoms, the patient denied any history of mania or hypomania. She described a history of frequent panic attacks in the past, with some accompanying agoraphobic avoidance, but said that these events had abated spontaneously 2

years ago. While she considers herself a "perfectionist," she denied frank obsessions or compulsions. There was no history of eating disorders, ADHD, somatization disorder, dissociative disorders, or psychotic phenomena. With regard to pesonality disorders, there was a hint of dependent traits in her description of her relationships with her husband and her best friend.

FAMILY HISTORY

If you draw a genogram directly on the evaluation form, this will suffice for the family psychiatric history, although you may want to add a one-line comment to highlight some facet of the history, such as

> The patient has a strong genetic loading for bipolar disorder, as shown in the genogram.

If you are dictating the evaluation, I suggest drawing a genogram on a blank sheet that you can staple to the back of the transcription, with the note "see attached genogram," in the family history section.

SOCIAL HISTORY

The thoroughness and length of the social history depend on clinician preference and the purpose of the evaluation. Obviously, a more lengthy social history is necessary in a psychotherapeutic evaluation than a psychopharmacologic evaluation. In addition, some clinical problems are more influenced by psychosocial issues than others. PTSD, for example, will always require a fairly extensive social history, whereas schizophrenia often develops independently of the social milieu.

At a minimum, your social history should include these pieces of information:

Where your patient was born and raised

Number of siblings

Birth order of patient and siblings

Who was present in the household during the formative years

Educational level

Work history

Marital and parenting history of patient

Typical daily activities other than work

The patient was born and raised in Lowell, Massachusetts, and is the youngest of three children, with a brother aged 50 and a sister aged 53. He describes his childhood as "normal" until his father died in a car accident when the patient was 10 years old, after which his mother was "always depressed." His grades in high school were Bs and Cs, and he went to technical school to study auto mechanics for 2 years. He eventually opened his own auto body business, which he still runs. He married his current wife, Diane, when he was 24, and they now have two children, both girls, ages 21 (Laura) and 24 (Angie). He is close to both of them. He works 6 days a week, and when he is not at work, he often watches television while drinking a beer and occasionally goes fishing with male friends. He described his relationship with his wife with the comment, "We get along."

MEDICAL HISTORY

You may use the mnemonic **MIDAS** to organize the medical history. I usually begin with a statement about the patient's general health, such as:

The patient reports that she is in good overall health.

The patient has suffered a number of chronic medical problems.

List any illnesses, surgeries, prescribed medications, and medication allergies. Note the name of the primary care physician. If you have asked questions from the medical review of systems, note any relevant answers. At a minimum, note whether the patient has had any seizures or head injuries, both of which are often germane to psychiatric problems.

The patient is in good general health and denies any history of major illnesses, surgeries, head injuries, or seizures. She takes no medications aside from birth control pills, and she reports an allergy to penicillin. She has regular gynecologic examinations with Dr. L.

The patient has a significant and complicated medical history, including heart disease, diabetes, and neurologic problems stemming from the diabetes. She had coronary bypass surgery last year. Currently, she has shortness of breath when she walks a half block, and she has constant pain in her feet. She recalls having had a concussion after falling off a horse when she was young, but she denies any seizure history. Her primary care physician is Dr. R, and her medications include insulin, captopril, Lasix, potassium supplement, Vicodin for pain, and Paxil (20 mg a day). She once had an allergic reaction to Wellbutrin, involving a total body rash.

MENTAL STATUS EXAMINATION

In writing up or dictating the mental status section of your diagnostic evaluation, temporarily shed your clinician's mantle and become a creative writer. Describe your patient so well that a reader would be able to recognize him from your description alone.

Compare the following two descriptions of the same patient:

> The patient was a 32-year-old man who was tired but cooperative with the interview. He was disheveled. Eye contact was good. Mood and affect were angry and irritable.

> The patient was interviewed in a medical bay of the emergency room. He was lying on his back on a gurney in four-point restraints, wearing a hospital gown. He had received 5 mg of Haldol intramuscularly shortly before the interview. As I walked in, he lifted his head and looked at me intensely, saying, "Will you get me the hell out of these shackles?" I assured him that I would do so if he posed no danger to himself or others. He was resigned and cooperative from that point on.

The second version gives a more vivid sense of the patient's mental status. Yes, he is angry and irritable, but this is in reaction to something in his environment. Furthermore, he's able to modulate his affect in response to the interviewer's statement, indicating a degree of control over his emotional state not communicated by the first summary. The "disheveled" of the first write-up might imply the self-neglect characteristic of schizophrenia, but in fact it's hard to look anything *but* disheveled when you're in a gurney with your limbs restrained.

That said, professional jargon *does* have its place in the write-up. This is especially true in the description of psychotic TP and TC. Words and phrases such as *tangentiality*, *looseness of associations*, and *ideas of reference* are technical terms with meanings that are understood throughout the mental health field, and they should be used when appropriate. The table below lists some common jargon-containing statements and some fresher alternatives.

Alternatives to jargon

Mental status jargon	More descriptive alternative
She was a cooperative informant.	She answered all questions in full but with a sense of apathy and indifference.
He was well-groomed.	He had short brown hair that was washed and combed, and he was clean-shaven.
She was disheveled.	She had long black hair that looked stiff and unwashed. Her hands were caked with dirt.
He showed psychomotor retardation; eye contact was poor.	He sat slumped over, staring at the floor, and was nearly motionless throughout the interview.
Speech was fluent and of low volume.	She spoke in a monotonous and wooden tone, and so softly that I had to lean toward her to understand her words.
Affect was flat and dysthymic.	He appeared sad and morose throughout the interview.

Your MSE can follow the format outlined in Chapter 19 (recall the mnemonic: All Borderline Subjects Are Tough, Troubled Characters). A good strategy is to limit jargon to those aspects of the MSE that are normal and to use more descriptive language for those parts of the examination that are directly relevant to the eventual diagnosis.

This was a well-groomed, pleasant-appearing woman, dressed in a professional suit and smelling strongly of perfume. She presented herself as serious and engaged. Her body was tense; she spoke rapidly and articulately as she related her psychiatric history. She seemed quite anxious, with her hands clenched around her billfold and her feet tapping the floor. Her stated mood was "I'm just barely holding on," and "I'm scared of having a panic attack all the time." Her TP was coherent in content and without hallucinations or delusions, but with some excessive rumination on the theme of getting "just the right medicine." She denied SI. On cognitive screen, concentration and memory were normal.

The patient presented as a somewhat disheveled man with long black hair, scraggly beard, and soiled clothes. He wore horn-rimmed glasses and had the look of an eccentric intellectual. He sat quietly for the most part and volunteered very little information; he seemed apathetic rather than guarded. His affect was bland, with a striking disparity between his stated mood ("I'm headed for a breakdown. I hate this life.") and his affect. His TP was coherent and without any LOA or flight of ideas. TC was impoverished. He denied any current hallucinations but admitted to having heard a voice calling his name "once or twice" over the preceding week. He said he wished he were dead but denied any plan to harm himself. On cognitive screen, concentration and memory were normal.

ASSESSMENT

The assessment should be a brief recapitulation of the over-all clinical picture and a discussion of differential diagnosis. Remember that many people who read your write-up will read only this section to get right to the point. Therefore, take pains to make the assessment both concise and informative.

This is a 27-year-old married, white, father of two who presents with a history consistent with bipolar disorder and a current clinical picture of major depression with NVSs of hypersomnia, lethargy, poor concentration, and increased appetite for sweet foods. In addition, he presents with significant anxiety, but he probably does not meet criteria for a discrete anxiety disorder, with the possible exception of GAD. Significant family conflict has contributed to his current illness.

This is a 52-year-old, never-married, African-American woman who has a long and complicated history of chronic mental illness, variously diagnosed as schizoaffective disorder and chronic schizophrenia. She presents now in a florid psychotic state with auditory hallucinations, ideas of reference, irritability, anxiety, and lack of sleep for 3 days. The current picture is confusing, and it may represent an irritable manic episode or an agitated depression with psychosis. Medication noncompliance may have been a precipitant, although chronic poverty is a relevant psychosocial factor.

DSM-IV DIAGNOSIS

It is important to list all five axes, realizing that insurance companies in particular rely heavily on this section in determining need for continuing care.

Axis I

Axis I refers to the main psychiatric diagnosis. While busy clinicians often get lazy in this section and write an unofficial or truncated diagnostic label, I suggest that you get into the habit early of making sure your diagnosis is actually listed as such in *DSM-IV*. The way to make sure you do this is to write down the *DSM-IV* code every time, an admittedly tedious (and, to some, clinically irrelevant) task. Writing down the code has the additional advantage of saving time later in the treatment when you request more treatment sessions and you have to write the *DSM-IV* code on the authorization request form.

To make this easier for you, I have included a pocket card in Appendix A with a list of the more common diagnoses and their *DSM* codes.

Axis II

The axis II section is where you code personality disorders and mental retardation. Because it is so hard to definitively diagnose a personality disorder after a single interview, it is common practice to either note a "rule out" diagnosis (e.g., "Rule out borderline personality disorder.") or to use the old standby, "personality disorder NOS," often specifying several candidate traits—for example, "Personality disorder NOS with borderline, histrionic, and narcissistic traits." One commonly sees "deferred" as the axis II diagnosis, which means that the clinician could not obtain enough information to decide whether a personality disorder existed. Although this may be the case, try not to use "deferred" too much, as it can turn into a cop-out from your clinical duty to actively probe for evidence of personality disorder traits.

Axis III

Note any general medical conditions that are significant, either in terms of contributing toward the psychiatric diagnosis (e.g., hypothyroidism aggravating depression) or affecting the patient's current functioning (e.g., heart disease, causing shortness of breath). You don't have to mention your patient's eczema or childhood tonsillectomy in this section, unless the problem is relevant.

Axis IV

The axis IV section is where you should note any psychosocial problems that may be aggravating the psychiatric condition or, in some cases, may be the result of it. *DSM-IV* groups these problems into nine helpful categories:

1. Problems with primary support group
2. Problems related to the social environment
3. Educational problems
4. Occupational problems
5. Housing problems
6. Economic problems
7. Problems with access to health care services
8. Problems related to interaction with the legal system
9. Other psychosocial and environmental problems

   Remember that some apparently positive events can contribute to psychiatric problems as well, as in the example of the patient who finally gets a big promotion and develops panic disorder related to fear of failure in the new position.

Axis V

The GAF is a numeric scale from 1 to 100 that indicates the degree to which the clinical disorder has impaired your patient's psychological, social, and occupational functioning. I consider it one of the more annoying contributions of the *DSM-IV* to the mental health care system, because the scores are subjective and vary widely among different practitioners. My GAF of 60 may be a colleague's GAF of 45. To make matters worse, most managed-care companies require you to note the GAF on treatment authorization forms, meaning that you have no choice but to learn the scale, no matter how useless you may find it to be.

Here's my own abbreviated "GAF-made-easy" scale that may facilitate your score-assignment chore.

GAF-made-easy scale

GAF score	Applicable clinical situation
90 and above	Probably none. Very few people with "absent or minimal symptoms" will make it into your office.
80	Patients who were once symptomatic but who have been successfully treated and are continuing to see you to maintain remission
70	*Mild* depression, mild anxiety, mild problems functioning
60	*Moderate* symptoms, moderate functioning problems
50	*Serious* symptoms, serious functioning problems
40	*Severe* symptoms. You will be considering hospitalization for patients with GAF of 40 or below.
30 and below	*Very severe* symptoms. If this patient is not yet in the hospital, call an ambulance immediately.

Rules of thumb:

1. In a typical outpatient mental health practice, patients will walk into your office with GAF scores of 50 or 60 and will improve to GAF scores of 70 or 80.
2. In a typical inpatient setting, patients are admitted with GAF scores of 40 or below and will be discharged with GAF scores of around 50.

TREATMENT PLAN

A good, concise treatment plan should include

- Any diagnostic testing planned (i.e., neuropsychological testing, laboratory tests)
- Plans for medication, if you can prescribe
- Plans for therapy, if needed
- Referrals to other health care practitioners, if applicable
- When you plan to see your patient again

For example,

> The plan is to obtain electrolytes, complete blood cell count, and thyroid panel to screen for organic causes of his symptoms; to start Zoloft at 25 mg per day, increasing to 50 mg per day, as tolerated (patient was informed of, and understood, potential risks and benefits of medication); and to start weekly cognitive behavioral therapy. I will see him again in 1 week.

> The plan is to begin psychodynamic therapy to address her grief issues and to refer to a psychiatrist for possible antianxiety medication. I will see her again in 1 week.

APPENDIXES

Psychiatric evaluation

Section of evaluation	Relevant data
Current complaint	
Source	
Identifying data/history of present illness	Chronology, precipitants, neuro-vegetative symptoms
Past psychiatric history	Go CHaMP
Suicidal ideation/suicide attempt	
Substances	Drug of choice, first use, last use, longest sobriety, detoxifications, history of seizure, delirium tremens
Legal history	
Psychiatric review of symptoms	Depression, mania, anxiety, psychosis, attention-deficit hyperactivity disorder, emotional disorder/disturbance, borderline, schizoid, antisocial
Past medical history	MIDAS, head trauma, brain studies, review of systems
Social history	Raised, abuse, education, work, relationships
Family history	
Mental status examination	Appearance, behavior, speech, mood, affect, thought process, thought content, cognitive
Physical examination	
Narrative assessment	
DSM-IV axes	
Plan	

(handwritten annotations in left margin: "All Borderlines ... objects Are Tough, Troubled ... or ...")

(handwritten annotation right of Mental status examination: "p. 116")

DSM-IV mnemonics

Major depression	**SIGECAPS** (4/8)
Dysthymia	**ACHEWS** (2/6)
Manic episode	**DIGFAST** (3/7)
Schizophrenia	**D**elusions **H**erald **S**chizophrenic's **B**ad **N**ews (2/5)
Substance abuse	**T**empted **W**ith **C**ognac (3/7)
Alcoholism	**CAGE** (2/4)
Panic attack	**H**eart (3)
	Breathlessness (5)
	Fear (5) (4/13)
Obsessive-compulsive disorder	**W**ashing and **S**traightening **M**ake **C**lean **H**ouses (1/5)
Posttraumatic stress disorder	**R**emembers (1) **A**trocious (3) **N**uclear (3) **A**ttacks (2)
Generalized anxiety disorder	**M**acbeth **F**rets **C**onstantly **R**egarding **I**llicit **S**ins (3/6)
Somatization disorder	**R**ecipe **4 P**ain: **C**onvert **2 S**tomachs to **1 S**ex (8/8)
Bulimia nervosa	**B**ulimics **O**ver**C**onsume **P**astries (4/4)
Anorexia nervosa	**W**eight **F**ear **B**others **A**norexics (4/4)
Dementia	Memory **BREW** (Memory + 1/4)
Delirium	Medical **FRAT** (5/5)
Attention-deficit hyperactivity disorder	**MOAT** (6/9)
Borderline personality disorder	**I DESPAIRR**

*The numbers in parentheses reflect the number of criteria required for diagnosis out of the total possible criteria.

Defense mechanisms

Mature defenses	Suppression
	Altruism
	Sublimation
	Humor
Neurotic defenses	Denial
	Repression
	Reaction formation
	Displacement
	Rationalization
Immature defenses	Passive aggression
	Acting out
	Dissociation
	Projection
	Splitting (idealization/devaluation)
Psychotic defenses	Denial of external reality
	Distortion of external reality

Appearance terms

Aspect	Appearance descriptors
Hair	Bald, thinning, close-cropped, short, long, shoulder-length, crew-cut, straight, curly, wavy, frizzy, braided, pony tail, pig tails, afro, relaxed, dreadlocks, unevenly cut, stiff, greasy, dry, matted
Facial hair	Clean-shaven, neatly trimmed beard, long scraggly beard, goatee, unshaven
Face	Attractive, nice-looking, pleasant, plain, pale, drawn, mongoloid, ruddy, flushed, bony, thin, broad, moon-shaped, red-nosed, thickly made-up
Eyes (gaze)	Good, shifty, averted, staring, fixated, dilated, downcast, forceful, intense, aggressive, piercing
Body	Thin, cachectic, lean, frail, underweight, normal build, muscular, husky, stocky, overweight, moderately obese, obese, morbidly obese, short, medium height, tall, tattooed arms
Movements	No abnormal movements, fidgety, bobbing knee, facial tic or twitch, lip-smacking, lip-puckering, tremulous, jittery, restless, wringing hands, motionless, rigid, limp, stiff, slumped
Clothes	Casually dressed, neat, appropriate, professional, immaculate, fashionable, sloppy, ill-fitting, outdated, flamboyant, sexually provocative, soiled, dirty, tight, loose, slogans on clothes

Affect terms

Affect	Terms
Normal	Appropriate, calm, pleasant, relaxed, normal, friendly, comfortable, unremarkable
Happy	Cheerful, bright, peppy, content, self-satisfied, silly, giggly, grandiose, euphoric, elated, exalted
Sad	Sad, gloomy, sullen, depressed, pessimistic, morose, hopeless, discouraged
Anxious	Anxious, worried, tense, nervous, apprehensive, frightened, terrified, bewildered, paranoid
Angry	Angry, irritable, disdainful, bitter, arrogant, defensive, sarcastic, annoyed, furious, enraged, hostile
Indifferent	Indifferent, shallow, superficial, cool, distant, apathetic, aloof, dull, vacant, affectless, uninterested, cynical

Rapid IQ test, Wilson Rapid Approximate Intelligence Test

Intelligence	Best effort	IQ
Retarded	2×6	<70
Borderline	2×24	70–80
Dull normal	2×48	80–90
Average	2×196	90–110

From I. C. Wilson (1967). Rapid approximate intelligence test. *Am J Psychiatry, 123*:1289–1290.

Heritability and prevalence of psychiatric disorders

DSM-IV disorder	Lifetime relative risk if first-degree relative has disorder[a]	Lifetime prevalence in general population[b]
Bipolar disorder	25	1
Schizophrenia	19	1
Bulimia nervosa	10	2[c]
Panic disorder	10	4
Alcoholism	7	14
Generalized anxiety disorder	6	5
Anorexia nervosa	5	1[c]
Simple phobia	3	11
Social phobia	3	13
Somatization disorder	3	2[d]
Major depression	3	17
Obsessive-compulsive disorder	?	3[e]
Agoraphobia	3	5

[a]Relative risk figures from R. O. Reider, C. Kaufmann, et al (1994). Genetics. In R. E. Hales, S. C. Yudofsky, and J. A. Talbott (Eds.), *American Psychiatric Press Textbook of Psychiatry.* Washington, DC: American Psychiatric Press. See Chapter 15, page 90, for explanation.

[b]Lifetime prevalence figures from R. C. Kessler, K. A. McGonagle, S. Zhao, et al. (1994). Lifetime and 12-month prevalence of *DSM-III-R* psychiatric disorders in the United States. *Archives of General Psychiatry, 51,* 8–19; and D. A. Regier, M. E. Farmer, et al. (1990). Comorbidity of mental disorders with alcohol and other drug abuse. *Journal of the American Medical Association, 264,* 2511–2518.

[c]From K. A. Halmi (1994). Eating disorders: anorexia nervosa, bulimia nervosa, and obesity. In R. E. Hales, S. C. Yudofsky, and J. A. Talbott (Eds.), *American Psychiatric Press Textbook of Psychiatry.* Washington, DC: American Psychiatric Press.

[d]From R. L. Martin and S. H. Yutzy (1994). Somatoform disorders. In R. E. Hales, S. C. Yudofsky, and J. A. Talbott (Eds.), *American Psychiatric Press Textbook of Psychiatry.* Washington, DC: American Psychiatric Press.

[e]From E. Hollander, D. Simeon, et al. (1994). Anxiety disorders. In R. E. Hales, S. C. Yudofsky, and J. A. Talbott (Eds.), *American Psychiatric Press Textbook of Psychiatry.* Washington, DC: American Psychiatric Press.

Weight table for women

Height	Ideal weight (lb, for medium frame)	15% under
4'10"	113	96
4'11"	115	98
5'0"	118	100
5'1"	121	103
5'2"	124	105
5'3"	127	108
5'4"	130	111
5'5"	133	113
5'6"	136	115
5'7"	139	118
5'8"	142	120
5'9"	145	123
5'10"	148	126
5'11"	151	128
6'0"	154	131

Weight table for men

Height	Ideal weight (lb, for medium frame)	15% under
5'2"	137	116
5'3"	139	118
5'4"	141	120
5'5"	143	122
5'6"	145	123
5'7"	148	126
5'8"	151	128
5'9"	154	131
5'10"	157	133
5'11"	160	136
6'0"	163	139
6'1"	167	142
6'2"	171	145
6'3"	175	149
6'4"	179	152

Common *DSM-IV* diagnoses

Diagnosis	Numeric code
Major depression, single episode, moderate	296.22
Major depression, recurrent, moderate	296.32
Dysthymic disorder	300.4
Bipolar I disorder, manic episode	296.42
Bipolar I disorder, depressed episode	296.52
Schizophrenia, paranoid type	295.30
Schizophrenia, undifferentiated type	295.90
Schizoaffective disorder	295.70
Alcohol dependence	303.90
Alcohol abuse	305.00
Polysubstance dependence	304.80
Panic disorder without agoraphobia	300.01
Panic disorder with agoraphobia	300.21
Social phobia	300.23
Obsessive-compulsive disorder	300.3
Posttraumatic stress disorder	309.81
Generalized anxiety disorder	300.02
Anxiety disorder NOS	300.00
Somatization disorder	300.81
Anorexia nervosa	307.1
Bulimia nervosa	307.51
Dementia of the Alzheimer's type, late onset, uncomplicated	290.0
Delirium	293.0
Attention-deficit hyperactivity disorder, combined type	314.01
Borderline personality disorder	301.83
Personality disorder NOS	301.9

GAF-made-easy scale

GAF score	Applicable clinical situation
90 and above	Probably none. Very few people with "absent or minimal symptoms" will make it into your office.
80	Patients who were once symptomatic, but who have been successfully treated and are continuing to see you to maintain remission.
70	*Mild* depression, mild anxiety, mild problems functioning.
60	*Moderate* symptoms, moderate functioning problems.
50	*Serious* symptoms, serious functioning problems.
40	*Severe* symptoms. You will consider hospitalization for patients with GAF of 40 or below.
30 and below	*Very severe* symptoms. If this patient is not yet in the hospital, call an ambulance immediately.

GAF, global assessment of functioning.

Mini–Mental State Examination

Orientation (score 1 point for correct response)
1. What is the year?
2. What is the season?
3. What is the date?
4. What is the day of the week?
5. What is the month?
6. Where are we? building or hospital?
7. Where are we? floor?
8. Where are we? town or city?
9. Where are we? county?
10. Where are we? state?

Registration (score 1 point for each object identified correctly, maximum is 3 points)
11. Name three objects at about one each second. Ask the patient to repeat them. If the patient misses an object, repeat them until all three are learned.

Attention and calculation (score 1 point for each correct answer up to maximum of 5 points)
12. Subtract 7s from 100 until 65 (or, as an alternative, spell "world" backwards).

Recall (score 1 point for each correct answer, maximum of 3)
13. Ask for names of three objects learned in question 11.

Language
14. Point to a pencil and a watch. Ask the patient to name each object. Score 1 point for each correct answer, maximum of 2 points.
15. Have the patient repeat "No ifs, ands, or buts." Score 1 point if correct.
16. Have the patient follow a three-stage command: "(1) Take the paper in your right hand. (2) Fold the paper in half. (3) Put the paper on the floor." Score 1 point for each command done correctly, maximum of 3 points.
17. Write the following in large letters: "CLOSE YOUR EYES." Ask the patient to read the command and perform the task. Score 1 point if correct.
18. Ask the patient to write a sentence of his or her own choice. Score 1 point if the sentence has a subject, an object, and a verb.

(*continued*)

Mini–Mental State Examination (*continued*)

19. Draw the design printed below. Ask the patient to copy the design. Score 1 point if all sides and angles are preserved and if the intersecting sides form a quadrangle.

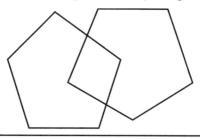

From M. F. Folstein, S. E. Folstein, and P. R. McHugh (1975). Mini-mental state. A practical method for grading the cognitive state of patients for the clinician. *Journal of Psychiatric Research 12*,189–198.

Age- and education-adjusted norms for the Folstein Mini–Mental State Examination (mean scores)

Education level (yr)	Age (yr)														
	18–24	25–29	30–34	35–39	40–44	45–49	50–54	55–59	60–64	65–69	70–74	75–79	80–84	≥85
0–4	22	25	25	23	23	23	23	22	23	22	22	21	20	19
5–8	27	27	26	26	27	26	27	26	26	26	26	25	24	23
9–12	29	29	29	28	28	28	28	28	28	28	27	27	25	26
College and higher	29	29	29	29	29	29	29	29	29	29	28	28	27	27

From R. M. Crum, J. C. Anthony, S. S. Bassett, and M. F. Folstein (1993). Population-based norms for the Mini–Mental State Examination by age and educational level. Journal of the American Medical Association, 269, 2386–2391.

Data Forms for the Interview

INITIAL PSYCHIATRIC EVALUATION (SHORT FORM)

Initial Psychiatric Evaluation
(Short Form)

Name: _____ Unit number: _____

Date: _____ Date of birth: _____

Insurance: _____

Contacts: _____

Current complaint/HPI:

_____
_____
_____

Past Psychiatric History   **Past Medical History**

Current treaters: Current medications:

_____   _____

Hospitalizations: Illnesses:

_____   _____

Medication trials: Surgeries:

_____   _____

Psychotherapy: Allergies:

_____   _____

Suicide attempts: Review of systems:
                                       head injury
_____
                                     _____
History violence/
  incarceration: Temporal lobe epilepsy:

_____   _____

Substance abuse:

_____

Family History

_____
_____
_____
_____

Social/Developmental History
Psychiatric review of systems

Depression   S   I   G   E   C   A   P   S

Mania   D   I   G   F   A   S   T

Anxiety disorder: agoraphobic, panic, obsessive-compulsive disorder, posttraumatic stress disorder, generalized anxiety disorder

Psychosis

Attention-deficit hyperactivity disorder, eating disorders

Personality

Mental Status Examination
A   B   S   A   T   T   C

Physical Examination

_____
_____
_____
_____
_____
_____

Laboratory Tests

_____
_____
_____
_____
_____
_____

INITIAL PSYCHIATRIC EVALUATION (LONG FORM)*

Initial Psychiatric Evaluation
(Long Form)

Name: _____ Referred by: _____
Date: _____ SSN: _____
Address: _____
Date of birth: _____ Occupation: _____
Phone: _____
Insurance: _____

Identifying Information
_____
_____

Presenting Symptoms
_____
_____

History of Present Illness
_____
_____

Past Psychiatric History
Hospitalizations: _____
Medication trials: _____
Psychotherapy: _____
Suicide attempts/gestures: _____
Legal history: _____

Substance Use History
Tobacco: _____
Caffeine: _____

---

*Adapted from the evaluation form of Anthony Erdmann, M.D.

Alcohol
   CAGE: _____
   Withdrawals: _____
   Adverse consequences: _____
   Last drink: _____
Marijuana: _____
Cocaine/other stimulants: _____
Opiates: _____
Benzodiazepines: _____
Hallucinogens: _____
Detoxification/rehabilitation: _____

Medical History
Primary care physician: _____
Current medications: _____
Illnesses: _____
Surgeries: _____
Drug allergies: _____

Medical Review of Systems
General: _____
Skin: _____
Head, ears, eyes, nose, and throat: _____
Cardiovascular and respiration: _____
Gastrointestinal: _____
Genitourinary/gynecology: _____
Neurology: _____

Family History (genogram)

Social History

_____

_____

Psychiatric Review of Symptoms

Depression: _____

Mania: _____

Suicidal ideation: _____

Psychosis/schizophrenia
- Symptoms (2/5, 1 month): ___delusions
  ___hallucinations ___disorganized speech
  ___disorganized/catatonic behavior
  ___negative symptoms
- Prodrome/residual (1/2, 6 months):
  ___negative symptoms
  ___2 positive symptoms

Anxiety
- GAD (3/6, 6 months): ___restless ___fatigue
  ___conscious ___irritable ___muscle tension
  ___insomnia
- Panic (4/13, recurrence + 1 month of worry):
  ___shortness of breath ___faint ___palpitations
  ___trembling ___sweating ___choking ___nauseous
  ___depersonalization/derealization
  ___numbness/tingling ___chest pain
  ___fear of dying ___fear of losing sanity
  ___chills/hot
- OCD: ___obsessions ___compulsions
  ___interfere/time conscious
- PTSD (1 month):
  Reexperience (1/5): ___memories ___dreams
  ___flashbacks ___distress/reexposure
  ___physiologic reactivity/reexposure
  Avoidance (3/7): ___thoughts/feelings
  ___activities/situations ___amnesia ___less interest
  ___estrangement ___restricted affect
  ___thought of no future
  Arousal (2/5): ___sleep ___irritability
  ___consciousness ___hypervigorous ___startle

- Social phobia (3/3): ___fear/social ___exposure/panic
  ___avoid/social

Cognitive
- Dementia:
  Memory problems
  Other cognitive problems (1/4): ___aphasia
  ___apraxia ___agnosia ___executive functions
- Delirium (5/5): ___disturb consciousness
  ___cognitive change ___short onset ___fluctuate
  ___medication/substance cause
- Attention-deficit hyperactivity disorder:
  Inattentive (6/9): ___details/mistakes ___attention
  ___listen ___follow through ___disorganized
  ___avoid/dislike mental effort ___loses things
  ___distract ___forgetful
  Hyperactive/impulsive (6/9): ___fidgets/squirms
  ___diff/seated ___runs/climbs ___blurts answers
  ___on/go/motor ___diff/play quietly
  ___talk excess ___interrupts/intrudes ___waits turn

Somatoform
- Somatization (3/7, starting before 30, lasting several
  years): ___shortness of breath ___dysmenorrhea
  ___burn sex organs ___lump/throat ___amnesia
  ___vomiting ___pain/extremities
- Anorexia (4/4): ___refuse/maintain weight
  ___fear of fat ___body distortion ___amenorrhea
- Bulimia (5/5): ___binge eating ___lack/control
  ___inappropriate weight/loss behavior
  ___>2 times/week for 3 months
  ___self-evaluation of body shape

Mental Status Examination

_____

_____

Neurovegetative symptoms

_____

_____

Cognitive Examination
- Orientation: _____
- Concentration: _____
- Memory tests:
  Three objects immediately
  Three objects at 3 minutes
  General information
    Presidents
    World War II
    Current news
  → Remote personal
    Date of wedding
    Name of high school/college

Assessment and Diagnostic Formulation

_____
_____

Axis I: _____
Axis II: _____
Axis III: _____
Axis IV: _____
Axis V: _____
  Current GAF: _____
  Past year highest GAF: _____
  Past year lowest GAF: _____

Treatment Plan
- Medications: _____
- Therapy: _____
- Follow-up: _____

PATIENT QUESTIONNAIRE*

Patient Questionnaire

Name: _____ Today's date: _____
Date of birth: _____
Address: _____
Telephone numbers
   Home: _____
   Work: _____
Occupation: _____
Insurance: _____

What is the main concern that led you to consult me?

_____
_____

When did it begin?

_____
_____

Psychiatric History

Outpatient Treatment

Have you ever had outpatient treatment for a psychiatric
disorder? _____
If yes, what was the disorder? _____

_____
_____

When and where did you receive treatment? _____

_____
_____

What type of treatment was it (e.g., psychotherapy, medication, behavior therapy, others)? _____

_____
_____
_____

What was the name of your therapist? _____
   Address: _____
   Phone: _____
Do you authorize me to communicate with your therapist?

_____

---

*Adapted from the questionnaire of Edward Messner, M.D.

Hospitalizations

Have you ever been hospitalized for a psychiatric disorder?

_____

If yes, what was the disorder, which hospital(s), and what were the dates? _____

_____

_____

Medication History

What medications are you taking now (medical or psychiatric)?

Drug	Dose	Frequency	Prescribing physician

What medications have you taken in the past?

Drug	Date	Reason for discontinuing

Do you use nonprescription medications? _____

If yes, which ones? _____

_____

_____

Do you or have you used recreational or illegal drugs?

_____

If yes, which drugs and how much?

_____

_____

Do you drink alcohol? _____

Are you concerned about how much you drink? _____

Are you annoyed at comments about your drinking? ___
Have you felt guilty about anything resulting from your
drinking? _____
Do you ever have a drink early in the day to calm your
nerves or get rid of a hangover? _____
Do you smoke? _____   If yes, what and how much?
_____

Beverages with caffeine:
Coffee _____ Tea _____ Cups per day _____
Colas _____ Others _____ Cans per day _____

Medical History

What illnesses or surgeries have you had in the past?
_____
_____
_____
_____
_____
_____

Do you have any illnesses at present? _____
If yes, please list:
_____
_____
_____
_____
_____

Have you ever had a head injury? _____
When? _____
_____
How did it occur? _____
Have you ever had an EEG or a CT scan of
  your head? _____
If yes, when, and what were the results? _____
_____

Name of your primary care physician: _____
  Address: _____
  Phone: _____
Do you authorize me to communicate with your
physician? _____

Brief Review of Symptoms

Symptoms or problem	No	Yes	Date began	Description
Frequent or severe headaches				
Dizziness/vertigo				
Convulsions or seizures				
Vision problems				
Hearing problems				
Smelling or taste problems				
Thyroid problems				
Cough/asthma				
Chest pain				
Shortness of breath				
Nausea/vomiting/ diarrhea				
Abdominal pain				
Constipation				
Urinary problems				
Arthritis				
Diabetes				
Walking problems				

Social History

Marital status: single _____ married _____
   widowed _____ divorced _____
If married, date of wedding: _____
   Spouse's date of birth: _____
   Spouse's occupation: _____
If widowed, date and cause of spouse's death: _____
_____
If divorced, date and reason for divorce: _____
_____

Children

Name   Age   Location

_____
_____
_____
_____

Others currently living in your household and their relationship to you:

Name   Relationship

_____
_____
_____
_____

Family Medical History

Mother's name: _____

Age: _____ If deceased, date and cause of death: _____

_____

Does (or did) she have any illnesses? _____

_____

Father's name: _____

Age: _____ If deceased, date and cause of death: _____

_____

Does (or did) he have any illnesses? _____

_____

Brothers and sisters:

Name   Age   Illnesses

_____
_____
_____
_____
_____

Family Psychiatric History

Has anyone in your family ever had a psychiatric disorder (e.g., depression, mania, schizophrenia, drug or alcohol abuse, anxiety problems, suicide attempts)? _____

If yes, please indicate nature of problem and the family member's relationship to you:

_____

_____

_____

_____

Have you ever been exposed to abuse? _____

If yes, was it physical? _____ sexual? _____

emotional? _____

Who was involved? _____

Educational History

	Name of school	Location	Dates
High school			
College			
Postgraduate			

Occupational History

Dates	Job titles	Reason job ended (if applicable)

Military service:

_____

_____

Adaptive History

What stresses have you overcome in the past?

_____

_____

_____

How did you do it?

_____

_____

_____

What was the best period of your life?

_____

_____

What are your personal strengths?

_____

_____

_____

Patient's signature: _____

Patient Education Handouts

MAJOR DEPRESSION*
Patient Information Handout

Who Gets Depressed?

Major depressive disorder, often referred to as clinical depression, is a common illness that can affect anyone. During any 1-year period, 17.6 million American adults, or 10% of the population, suffer from either a major or minor depression.

What Is Depression?

Depression is not just "feeling blue" or being "down in the dumps." It is more than being sad or feeling grief after a loss. Depression is an illness (in the same way that diabetes, high blood pressure, and heart disease are illnesses) that affects your thoughts, feelings, physical health, and behaviors day after day.

Depression may be caused by many things, including the following:

- stressful or depressing life events
- family history and genetics
- certain medical illnesses
- certain medicines
- drugs or alcohol
- other psychiatric conditions

Certain life conditions (e.g., extreme stress or grief), may bring on a depression or prevent a full recovery. In some people, depression occurs even when life is going well. Depression is not your fault, nor is it a weakness. It is an illness, and it is treatable.

---

*This handout was adapted from public domain information supplied by both the National Institute of Mental Health and the Agency for Health Care Policy and Research (an agency of the U.S. Public Health Service).

How Will I Know Whether I Am Depressed?

People who have major depressive disorder have a number of symptoms nearly every day, all day, for at least 2 weeks. These always include at least one of the following:

- loss of interest in things you used to enjoy
- feeling sad, blue, or down in the dumps

You may also have at least three of the following symptoms:

- feeling slowed down or restless and unable to sit still
- feeling worthless or guilty
- increase or decrease in appetite or weight
- thoughts of death or suicide
- problems concentrating, thinking, remembering, or making decisions
- trouble sleeping or sleeping too much
- loss of energy or feeling tired all of the time

With depression, other physical or psychological symptoms are often present, including the following:

- headaches
- other aches and pains
- digestive problems
- sexual problems
- feeling pessimistic or hopeless
- being anxious or worried

How Is Depression Treated?

Depression is treated with either psychotherapy (counseling), medications, or both treatments combined.

Psychotherapy. The most effective psychotherapies for depression are

1. Cognitive therapy, in which the therapist points out ways that your thinking is negative and may actually cause you to be more depressed.
2. Interpersonal therapy, in which the focus is on improving the quality of your relationships with important people in your life.

Psychotherapy may take one to several months to cure your depression.

Medications. Many effective medications for depression exist. The most commonly prescribed are the selective serotonin reuptake inhibitors (SSRIs), which have names like Prozac, Zoloft, Paxil, and Luvox. These are popular because they have very few side effects when compared with older medications.

When someone begins taking an antidepressant, improvement generally will not begin to show immediately. With most of these medications, it will take from 1 to 3 weeks before changes begin to occur. Some symptoms diminish early in treatment; others, later. For instance, a person's energy level or his sleeping or eating patterns may improve before his depressed mood lifts. If there is little or no change in symptoms after 5 to 6 weeks, a different medication may be tried. Some people will respond better to one than to another. Because there is no way of determining beforehand which medication will be effective, the doctor may have to prescribe first one, then another, until an effective medication is found. Treatment is continued for a minimum of several months and may last up to a year or more.

BIPOLAR DISORDER*
Patient Information Handout

What Is Bipolar Disorder?

Bipolar disorder, which is also known as manic-depressive illness, is a mental illness involving episodes of serious mania and depression. The person's mood usually swings from overly high and irritable to sad and hopeless, and then back again, with periods of normal mood in between. Bipolar disorder typically begins in adolescence or early adulthood and continues throughout life. At least 2 million Americans suffer from manic-depressive illness. Bipolar disorder tends to run in families and is believed to be inherited in many cases.

Key Features of Bipolar Disorder

Bipolar disorder involves cycles of mania and depression. Signs and symptoms of **mania** include discrete periods of

- increased energy, activity, restlessness, racing thoughts, and rapid talking
- excessive high or euphoric feelings
- extreme irritability and distractibility
- decreased need for sleep
- unrealistic beliefs in one's abilities and powers
- uncharacteristically poor judgment
- a sustained period of behavior that is different from usual
- increased sexual drive
- abuse of drugs, particularly cocaine, alcohol, and sleeping medications
- provocative, intrusive, or aggressive behavior
- denial that anything is wrong

Signs and symptoms of **depression** include discrete periods of

- persistent sad, anxious, or empty mood
- feelings of hopelessness or pessimism
- feelings of guilt, worthlessness, or helplessness
- loss of interest or pleasure in ordinary activities, including sex
- decreased energy, a feeling of fatigue or of being "slowed down"

---

*This handout was adapted from public domain information supplied by the National Institute of Mental Health.

- difficulty concentrating, remembering, making decisions
- restlessness or irritability
- sleep disturbances
- loss of appetite and weight, or weight gain
- chronic pain or other persistent bodily symptoms that are not caused by physical disease
- thoughts of death or suicide; suicide attempts

How Is It Treated?

The most effective treatment for bipolar disorder is one of a variety of mood-stabilizing medications. The most well-known of these is **lithium**, which was the first medication introduced for bipolar disorder. More recently, two other medications have been introduced: **Tegretol** and **Depakote**. Although all medications for bipolar disorder are effective, side effects, including sedation, weight gain, and light-headedness, often occur. Psychiatrists can minimize these side effects by adjusting the dosage and formulation of medications.

In addition to medications, psychotherapy is helpful, especially during the depressed phase of bipolar disorder. Combination treatment (medications in combination with therapy) leads to the best results for most patients.

PANIC DISORDER*
Patient Information Handout

— "It started 10 years ago. I was sitting in a seminar in a hotel and this thing came out of the clear blue. I felt like I was dying."

— "For me, a panic attack is almost a violent experience. I feel like I'm going insane. It makes me feel like I'm losing control in a very extreme way. My heart pounds really hard, things seem unreal, and there's this very strong feeling of impending doom."

— "Between attacks there is this dread and anxiety that it's going to happen again. It can be very debilitating, trying to escape those feelings of panic."

What Is Panic Disorder?

People with panic disorder have feelings of terror that strike suddenly and repeatedly with no warning. They can't predict when an attack will occur, and many develop intense anxiety between episodes, worrying when and where the next one will strike. Between episodes they feel a persistent, lingering worry that another attack could come any minute. When a panic attack strikes, your heart most likely pounds, and you may feel sweaty, weak, faint, or dizzy. Your hands may tingle or feel numb, and you might feel flushed or chilled. You may have chest pain or smothering sensations, a sense of unreality, or fear of impending doom or loss of control. You may genuinely believe you're having a heart attack or stroke, losing your mind, or on the verge of death. Attacks can occur any time, even during nondream sleep. Most attacks average a couple of minutes, but occasionally they can go on for up to 10 minutes. In rare cases, they may last an hour or more.

Panic disorder is often accompanied by other conditions, such as depression or alcoholism, and may spawn phobias, which can develop in places or situations where panic attacks have occurred. For example, if a panic attack strikes while you're riding an elevator, you may develop a fear of elevators and start avoiding them. Some people's lives become greatly

---

*This handout was adapted from public domain information supplied by both the National Institutes of Health and the National Institute of Mental Health.

restricted—they avoid normal, everyday activities such as grocery shopping, driving, or even leaving the house. They may be able to confront a feared situation only if accompanied by a spouse or other trusted person. Basically, they avoid any situation they fear would make them feel helpless if a panic attack occurred. When people's lives become so restricted by the disorder, as happens in about one-third of all people with panic disorder, the condition is called *agoraphobia*. A tendency toward panic disorder and agoraphobia runs in families. Nevertheless, early treatment of panic disorder can often stop the progression to agoraphobia.

Panic attack symptoms
- Pounding heart
- Chest pains
- Lightheadedness or dizziness
- Nausea or stomach problems
- Flushes or chills
- Shortness of breath, or a feeling of smothering or choking
- Tingling or numbness
- Shaking or trembling
- Feelings of unreality
- Terror
- A feeling of being out of control or going crazy
- Fear of dying
- Sweating

Who Gets Panic Disorder?

Panic disorder strikes at least 1.6% of the population and is twice as common in women as in men. It can appear at any age, but most often it begins in young adults. Not everyone who experiences panic attacks will develop panic disorder—for example, many people have one attack but never have another. For those who do have panic disorder, though, it's important to seek treatment.

How Is Panic Disorder Treated?

Studies have shown that proper treatment—a type of psychotherapy called cognitive-behavioral therapy, medications, or possibly a combination of the two—helps 70% to 90% of people with panic disorder. Significant improvement is usually seen within 6 to 8 weeks. Cognitive-behavioral approaches teach patients how to view the panic situations differently and demonstrate ways to reduce anxiety (e.g., using breathing exercises or techniques to refocus attention). *Exposure therapy,* a technique used in cognitive-behavioral therapy, often helps to alleviate the phobias that may result from panic disorder. In exposure therapy, people are very slowly exposed to the fearful situation until they become desensitized to it. Some people find the greatest relief from panic disorder symptoms when they take certain prescription medications. Such medications, like cognitive-behavioral therapy, can help to prevent panic attacks or reduce their frequency and severity. Two types of medications that have been shown to be safe and effective in the treatment of panic disorder are antidepressants and benzodiazepines.

OBSESSIVE-COMPULSIVE DISORDER*
Patient Information Handout

What Is Obsessive-Compulsive Disorder?

Obsessive-compulsive disorder (OCD), one of the anxiety disorders, is a potentially disabling condition that can persist throughout a person's life. The individual who suffers from OCD becomes trapped in a pattern of repetitive thoughts and behaviors that are senseless and distressing but extremely difficult to overcome. OCD occurs in a spectrum from mild to severe; if severe and untreated, it can destroy a person's capacity to function at work, school, or even home.

How Common Is Obsessive-Compulsive Disorder?

For many years, mental health professionals thought of OCD as a rare disease, because only a minority of their patients had the condition. The disorder often went unrecognized because many of those afflicted with OCD, in efforts to keep their repetitive thoughts and behaviors secret, failed to seek treatment. However, a survey conducted in the early 1980s by the National Institute of Mental Health showed that OCD affects more than 2% of the population, making it more common than such severe mental illnesses as schizophrenia, bipolar disorder, or panic disorder. OCD strikes people of all ethnic groups. Men and women are equally affected.

Key Features of Obsessive-Compulsive Disorder

Obsessions.   *Obsessions* are unwanted ideas or impulses that repeatedly well up in the mind of the person with OCD. Common are persistent fears that harm may come to self or a loved one, an unreasonable concern with becoming contaminated, or an excessive need to do things correctly or perfectly. Again and again, the individual experiences a disturbing thought, such as, "My hands may be contaminated—I must wash them," "I may have left the gas on," or "I am going to injure my child." These thoughts are intrusive, unpleasant, and

---

*This handout was adapted from public domain information supplied by the National Institute of Mental Health.

produce a high degree of anxiety. Sometimes the obsessions are of a violent or a sexual nature, or they concern illness.

Compulsions.   In response to their obsessions, most people with OCD resort to repetitive behaviors called *compulsions*. The most common of these are washing and checking. Other compulsive behaviors include counting (often while performing another compulsive action such as hand-washing), repeating, hoarding, and endlessly rearranging objects in an effort to keep them in precise alignment. Mental problems, such as mentally repeating phrases, making lists, or checking are also common. These behaviors generally are intended to ward off harm to self or others. Some people with OCD have regimented rituals; others have rituals that are complex and changing. Performing rituals may give the person with OCD some relief from anxiety, but it is only temporary.

How Is Obsessive-Compulsive Disorder Treated?   OCD
is treated with either psychotherapy (counseling), medications, or both treatments combined.

PSYCHOTHERAPY
The most effective psychotherapy for OCD is cognitive-behavioral therapy. In this technique, your therapist will have you practice exposing yourself to those situations that make you anxious and cause you to act out a compulsion (such as checking or washing). Your therapist will help you to prevent the OCD response. Some of the exposure is done in the therapist's office, but most of it is done at home and is assigned as "homework."

Cognitive-behavioral therapy is very effective, especially for those patients who suffer primarily from compulsions. In such patients, therapy is often more effective than medication.

MEDICATIONS
Many effective medications for OCD exist. The most commonly prescribed are the selective serotonin reuptake inhibitors (SSRIs), which have names like Prozac, Zoloft, Paxil, and Luvox. These are popular because they have very few side effects when compared with older medications. Another effective medication is Anafranil, which tends to have more side effects than the SSRIs.

When someone begins taking an OCD medication, improvement generally will not begin to show immediately. With most of these medications, it takes from 1 to 3 weeks before changes begin to occur. If there is little or no change in symptoms after 5 to 6 weeks, a different medication may be tried. Because there is no way of determining beforehand which medication will be effective, the doctor may have to prescribe first one, then another, until an effective medication is found. Treatment is continued for a minimum of several months and may last up to a year or more.

References

Ainslie, N. K., and Murden, R. A. (1993). Effect of education on the clock-drawing dementia screen in non-demented elderly persons. *Journal of the American Geriatric Society, 41,* 249–252.

Andreasen, N. C. (1979). Thought, language, and communication disorders. I. Clinical assessment, definition of terms, and evaluation of their reliability. *Archives of General Psychiatry, 36,* 1315–1321.

Andreasen, N. C. (1982). Negative symptoms in schizophrenia: Definition and reliability. *Archives of General Psychiatry, 39,* 784–788.

Andreasen, N. J., Tsuang, M. T., and Canter, A. (1974). The significance of thought disorder in diagnostic evaluations. *Comprehensive Psychiatry, 15,* 27–34.

Anthony, J. C., LeResche, L., Niaz, U., von Korff, M.R., and Folstein, M.F. (1982). Limits of the mini-mental state as a screening test for dementia and delirium among hospital patients. *Psychological Medicine, 12,* 397–408.

Asnis, G. M., Kaplan, M. L., van Praag, H. M., and Sanderson, W. C. (1994). Homicidal behaviors among psychiatric outpatients. *Hospital and Community Psychiatry, 45,* 127–132.

Azar, B. (January 1997). Poor recall mars research and treatment. *APA Monitor,* p. 1.

Baekeland, F., and Lundwall, L. (1975). Dropping out of treatment: A critical review. *Psychological Bulletin, 82,* 738–783.

Barlow, D. (Ed.). (1993). *Clinical handbook of psychological disorders.* New York: The Guilford Press.

Beckman, H. B., and Franckel, R. M. (1984). The effect of physician behavior on the collection of data. *Annals of Internal Medicine, 101,* 692–696.

Biederman, J. (1991). Attention deficit hyperactivity disorder (ADHD). *Annals of Clinical Psychiatry, 3,* 9–22.

Binder, R. L., and McNiel, D. E. (1996). Application of the Tarasoff ruling and its effect on the victim and the therapeutic relationship. *Psychiatric Services, 47,* 1212–1215.

Blacker, D., and Tsuang, M. T. (1992). Contested boundaries of bipolar disorder and the limits of categorical diagnosis in psychiatry. *American Journal of Psychiatry, 149,* 1473–1483.

Boyd, J. H. (1986). Use of mental health services for the treatment of panic disorder. *American Journal of Psychiatry, 143,* 1569–1574.

Burke, J. D., Jr., and Regier, D. A. (1994) Epidemiology of mental disorders. In R. E. Hales, S. C. Yudofsky, and J. A. Talbott (Eds.), *American Psychiatric Press Textbook of Psychiatry.* Washington, DC: American Psychiatric Press.

Carlat, D. J., Camargo, C. A., Jr., and Herzog, D. B. (1997). Eating disorders in males: A report on 135 patients. *American Journal of Psychiatry, 154,* 1127–1132.

Chochinov, H. M., Wilson, K. G., Enns, M., and Lander, S. (1997). Are you depressed? Screening for depression in the terminally ill. *American Journal of Psychiatry, 154,* 674–676.

Clark, D. C., and Fawcett, J. (1992). An empirically based model of suicide risk assessment for patients with affective disorders. In D. Jacobs (Ed.), *Suicide and Clinical Practice.* Washington, DC: American Psychiatric Press.

Clark, W. D. (1981). Alcoholism: Blocks to diagnosis and treatment. *American Journal of Medicine, 71,* 275–288.

Cox, A., Holbrook, D., and Rutter, M. (1981). Psychiatric interviewing techniques. VI. Experimental study: Eliciting feelings. *British Journal of Psychiatry, 139,* 144–152.

Cox, A., Hopkinson, K., and Rutter, M. (1981). Psychiatric interviewing techniques. II. Naturalistic study: Eliciting factual information. *British Journal of Psychiatry, 138,* 283–291.

Cox, A., Rutter, M., and Holbrook, D. (1988). Psychiatric interviewing techniques. A second experimental study: Eliciting feelings. *British Journal of Psychiatry, 152,* 64–72.

Crook, T., Ferris, S., McCarthy, M., and Rae, D. (1980). Utility of digit recall tasks for assessing memory in the aged. *Journal of Consulting and Clinical Psychology, 48,* 228–233.

Eisenthal, S., Emery, R., Lazare, A., and Udin, H. (1979). "Adherence" and the negotiated approach to patienthood. *Archives of General Psychiatry, 36,* 393–398.

Elstein, A. S., Shulman, L. S., and Sprafka, S. A. (1978). *Medical Problem-Solving: An Analysis of Clinical Reasoning.* Cambridge, MA: Harvard University Press.

Ewing, J. A. (1984). Detecting alcoholism. The CAGE questionnaire. *Journal of the American Medical Association, 252,* 1905–1907.

Felthous, A. R. (1991). Duty to warn or protect: Current status for psychiatrists. *Psychiatric Annals, 21,* 591–598.

First, M., Frances, A., and Pincus, H. A. (1995). *DSM-IV Handbook of Differential Diagnosis.* Washington, DC: American Psychiatric Press.

Flaum, M. (1995). The diagnosis of schizophrenia. In C. Shriqui and H. Nasrallah (Eds.), *Contemporary Issues in the Treatment of Schizophrenia.* Washington, DC: American Psychiatric Press Inc.

Folstein, M. F., Folstein, S. E., and McHugh, P. R. (1975). "Mini-mental state." A practical method for grading the cognitive state of patients for the clinician. *Journal of Psychiatric Research, 12,* 189–198.

Frank, E., Kupfer, D. J., and Siegel, L. R. (1995). Alliance not compliance: A philosophy of outpatient care. *Journal of Clinical Psychiatry, 56* (suppl 1), 11–16.

Frank, J. D., and Frank, J. B. (1991). *Persuasion and Healing.* Baltimore, MD: The Johns Hopkins University Press.

Hall, R. C., Gardner, E. R., Stickney, S. K., LeCann, A. F., and Popkin, M. K. (1980). Physical illness manifesting as psychiatric disease. II. Analysis of a state hospital inpatient population. *Archives of General Psychiatry*, 37, 989–995.

Halmi, K. A. (1994). Eating disorders: Anorexia nervosa, bulimia nervosa, and obesity. In R. E. Hales, S. C. Yudofsky, and J. A. Talbott (Eds.), *American Psychiatric Press Textbook of Psychiatry*. Washington, DC: American Psychiatric Press.

Harwood, D. M., Jr., Hope, T., and Jacoby, R. (1997). Cognitive impairment in medical inpatients. I. Screening for dementia—is history better than mental state? *Age and Ageing*, 26, 31–35.

Havens, L. (1986). *Making Contact*. Cambridge, MA: Harvard University Press.

Havens, L. (1989). *A Safe Place*. New York: Random House.

Hinton, J., and Withers, E. (1971). The usefulness of clinical tests of the sensorium. *British Journal of Psychiatry*, 119, 9–18.

Hollander, E., Simeon, D., and Gorman, J. M. (1994). Anxiety disorders. In R. E. Hales, S. C. Yudofsky, and J. A. Talbott (Eds.), *American Psychiatric Press Textbook of Psychiatry*. Washington, DC: American Psychiatric Press.

Isaacs, B., and Kennie, A. (1973). The set test as an aid to the detection of dementia in old people. *British Journal of Psychiatry*, 123, 467–470.

Jacobs, M., Frank, E., Kupfer, D. J., Cornes, C., and Carpenter, L. L. (1987). A psychoeducational workshop for depressed patients, family, and friends: Description and evaluation. *Hospital and Community Psychiatry*, 38, 968–972.

Jorm, A., Scott, R., Cullen, J. S., and MacKinnon, A. J. (1991). Performance of the Informant Questionnaire on Cognitive Decline in the Elderly (IQCODE) as a screening test for dementia. *Psychological Medicine*, 21, 785–790.

Kaplan, C. (1995). Hypothesis testing. In M. J. Lipkin, S. M. Putnam, and A. Lazare (Eds.), *The Medical Interview*. New York: Springer-Verlag.

Keller, M. B., and Manschreck, T. C. (1989). The mental status examination. II. Higher intellectual functioning. In A. Lazare (Ed.), *Outpatient Psychiatry: Diagnosis and Treatment*. Baltimore, MD: Williams & Wilkins.

Kessler, R. C., McGonagle, K. A., Zhao, S., Nelson, C. B., Hughes, M., Eshleman, S., Wittchen, H. U., and Kendler, K. S. (1994). Lifetime and 12-month prevalence of DSM-III-R psychiatric disorders in the United States. *Archives of General Psychiatry*, 51, 8–19.

Klein, D. N., Riso, L. P., and Anderson, R. L. (1993). DSM-III-R dysthymia: Antecedents and underlying assumptions. *Progress in Experimental Perspectives in Psychopathologic Research*, 16, 222–253.

Lazare, A., Eisenthal, S., and Wasserman, L. (1975). The customer approach to patienthood—attending to patient requests in a walk-in clinic. *Archives of General Psychiatry, 32,* 553–558.

Lejoyeux, M., Ades, J., Tassain, V., and Solomon, J. (1997). Phenomenology and psychopathology of uncontrolled buying. *American Journal of Psychiatry, 153,* 1524–1529.

Lipkin, M. L. (1987). The medical interview and related skills. In W. T. Branch, Jr. (Ed.), *Office Practice of Medicine* (pp. 1287–1306). Philadelphia: W. B. Saunders.

Lishman, W. A. (1987). *Organic Psychiatry.* Boston: Blackwell Scientific.

Martin, R. L., and Yutzy, S. H. (1994). Somatoform disorders. In R. E. Hales, S. C. Yudofsky, and J. A. Talbott (Eds.), *American Psychiatric Press Textbook of Psychiatry.* Washington, DC: American Psychiatric Press.

McKenna, P. J. (1994). *Schizophrenia and Related Syndromes.* Oxford, UK: Oxford University Press.

Miller, G. A. (1957). The magical number seven, plus or minus: Some limits on our capacity for processing information. *Psychological Review, 63,* 81–97.

Milstein, V., Small, J. G., and Small, I. F. (1972). The subtraction of serial sevens test in psychiatric patients. *Archives of General Psychiatry, 26,* 439–441.

Morrison, J. (1995). *The First Interview.* New York: The Guilford Press.

Morrison, J., and Munoz, R. A. (1991). *Boarding Time: A Psychiatry Candidate's Guide to Part II of the ABPN Examination.* Washington, DC: American Psychiatric Press.

Murden, R. A., McRae, T. D., Kaner, S., and Bucknam, M. E. (1991). Mini-mental state exam scores vary with education in blacks and whites. *Journal of the American Geriatric Society, 39,* 149–155.

Norton, G. R., Dorward, J., and Cox, B. J. (1986). Factors associated with panic attacks in nonclinical subjects. *Behavior Therapy, 17,* 239–252.

Othmer, E., and Othmer, S. C. (1994). *The Clinical Interview Using DSM-IV.* Washington, DC: American Psychiatric Press.

Patterson, W. M., Dohn, H. H., Bird, J., and Patterson, G. (1983). Evaluation of suicidal patients: The SAD PERSONS scale. *Psychosomatics, 24,* 343–349.

Payne, S. L. (1951). *The Art of Asking Questions.* Princeton, NJ: Princeton University Press.

Pekarik, G. (1993). Beyond effectiveness: Uses of consumer-oriented criteria in defining treatment success. In T. Giles (Ed.), *Handbook of Effective Psychotherapy.* New York: Plenum Press.

Pilowsky, I., and Boulton, D. M. (1970). Development of a questionnaire-based decision rule for classifying depressed patients. *British Journal of Psychiatry, 116,* 647–650.

Pinkofsky, H. B. (1997). Mnemonics for DSM-IV personality disorders. *Psychiatric Services*, 48, 1197–1198.

Platt, F. W., and McMath, J. C. (1979). Clinical hypocompetence: The interview. *Annals of Internal Medicine*, 91, 898–902.

Rapp, M. S. (1979). Re-examination of the clinical mental status examination. *Canadian Journal of Psychiatry*, 24, 773–775.

Regier, D. A., Farmer, M. E., Rae, D. S., et al. (1990). Comorbidity of mental disorders with alcohol and other drug abuse. *Journal of the American Medical Association*, 264, 2511–2518.

Reider, R. O., Kaufmann, C. A., and Knowles, J. A. (1994). Genetics. In R. E. Hales, S. C. Yudofsky, and J. A. Talbott (Eds.), *American Psychiatric Press Textbook of Psychiatry*. Washington, DC: American Psychiatric Press.

Sacks, M. H., Carpenter, W. T., Jr., and Strauss, J. S. (1974). Recovery from delusions. Three phases documented by patient's interpretation of research procedures. *Archives of General Psychiatry*, 30, 117–120.

Searight, H. R., Nahlik, J. E., and Campbell, D. C. (1995). Attention-deficit/hyperactivity disorder: Assessment, diagnosis, and management. *The Journal of Family Practice*, 40, 270–279.

Shea, S. C. (1988). *Psychiatric Interviewing: The Art of Understanding*. Philadelphia: W. B. Saunders.

Smith, A. (1967). The serial sevens subtraction test. *Archives of Neurology*, 17, 78–80.

Solomon, S. D., and Davidson, J. R. T. (1997). Trauma: Prevalence, impairment, service use, and cost. *Journal of Clinical Psychiatry*, 58 (suppl 9), 5–11.

Steinweg, D. L., and Worth, H. (1993). Alcoholism: The keys to the CAGE. *The American Journal of Medicine*, 94, 520–523.

Stunkard, A. J., Fernstrom, M. H., Price, A., et al. (1990). Direction of weight change in recurrent depression. *Archives of General Psychiatry*, 47, 857–860.

Sudman, S., and Bradburn, N. M. (1987). *Asking Questions: A Practical Guide to Questionnaire Design*. San Francisco: Jossey-Bass.

Sullivan, H. S. (1970). *The Psychiatric Interview*. New York: W. W. Norton and Co.

Tangalos, E. G., Smith, G. E., Ivnik, R. J., Petersen, R. C., Kokmen, E., Kurland, L. T., Offord, K. P., and Parisi, J. E. (1996). The mini-mental state examination in general medical practice: Clinical utility and acceptance. *Mayo Clinic Proceedings*, 71, 829–837.

Tardiff, K. (1992). The current state of psychiatry in the treatment of violent patients. *Archives of General Psychiatry*, 49, 493–499.

Tolle, R., and Goetze, V. (1987). On the daily rhythm of depressive symptomology. *Psychopathology*, 20, 237–249.

Turner, C. F., Ku, L., Sonenstein, F. L., and Pleck, J. H. (1996). Impact of audio-CASI on bias in reporting of male-male sexual contacts. In R. B. Warnecke (Ed.), *Health Survey Research Methods*. Hyattsville, MD: National Center for Health Statistics.

Vaillant, G. E. (1988). Defense Mechanisms. In A. M. Nicholi, Jr. (Ed.), *The New Harvard Guide to Psychiatry*. Cambridge, MA: Harvard University Press.

Weissenburger, J., Rush, A. J., Giles, D. E., and Stunkard, A. J. (1986). Weight change in depression. *Psychiatry Research*, *17*, 275–283.

Wilson, I. C. (1967). Rapid approximate intelligence test. *American Journal of Psychiatry*, *123*, 1289–1290.

Winokur, G. (1981). *Depression: The Facts*. Oxford, UK: Oxford University Press.

Index